Mediterranean Diet for Beginners

The Complete Guide and 30-Day Meal Plan with 100 Healthy Mediterranean Diet Recipes for Weight Loss

Bryan Coleman

ISBN-13: 978- 1075189920

DEDICATION

To all who desire to live life to the fullest!

TABLE OF CONTENT

INTRODUCTION

The Greeks and Italians benefitted from whole foods and physical activity that made them less susceptible to diseases and remarkably healthier compared to other people. Research shows that the Mediterranean diet is associated with weight loss, long life, lower susceptibility to Alzheimer's and Parkinson's diseases, decreased risk of heart diseases, lower cholesterol, prevention of type II diabetes, strokes and heart attacks. Also, the Mediterranean diet also decreases the risk of anxiety, depression and certain cancers.

The Mediterranean diet is based on the long-established customary foods of the countries bordering the Mediterranean Sea. The origin of this phenomenal diet dates back to as early as the 1960s. Instead of a strict plan or a finite rule, it is a lifestyle that stresses the consumption of whole foods and the need for physical activity. The Mediterranean diet lays emphasis on the consumption of fish, legumes, whole grains, veggies, fruits and olive oil. Poultry and eggs can be eaten infrequently, but then again processed foods and red meats should be avoided as much as possible. Moderate amounts of fermented diary can be consumed on a regular basis, in addition, red wine should be consumed responsibly.

The Mediterranean Diet for Beginners contains a comprehensive guide to the Mediterranean diet and 100 delicious recipes for weight loss and a healthy life. This book will serve as a kick-start guide to help you get started on the Mediterranean diet to suit your preferences and specific wants. You will discover a diet that will help you make little or major changes towards a healthier life. The recipes in this book includes complete nutritional information to guide you as you cook your way to health. Also, this section contains a 30-day meal plan. Feel free to modify your food choices and portions based on your own preferences and needs.

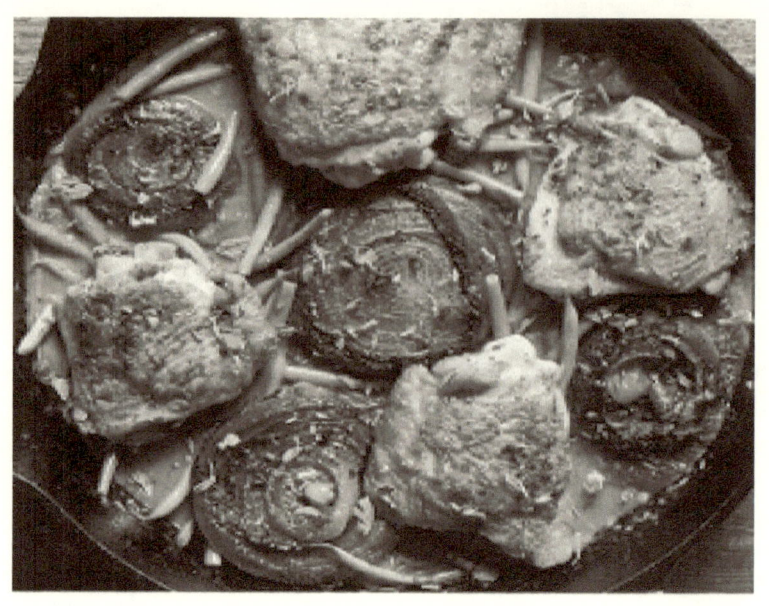

KICKSTART GUIDE

The Mediterranean diet is a straightforward diet with a simple approach. The concept is to copy the way of eating of the Mediterranean people. When uncertain, a simple formula to follow on the diet is to make a quarter of your plate - healthy protein, a quarter of your plate - whole grains, and the remaining half of your plate - vegetables and fruits. That is to say, a Mediterranean diet plate is divided into 3 parts (1/4 healthy protein, 1/4 whole grains and 1/2 veggies and fruits).

Here are some extra tips to get you started:

Avoid Processed Foods

Whole foods such as fish, legumes, nuts, whole grains, veggies, fruits and olive oil are the core of the Mediterranean diet. Consume whole foods that are beneficial to your body and health, and steer clear of processed foods to avoid violating the healthy principles of the Mediterranean diet.

Eat Fish Instead of Red Meat

The major supply of protein on the Mediterranean diet are fatty fish such as herring, tuna, mackerel and salmon. These fish are loaded with astronomical amounts of omega-3 fatty acids which improves cholesterol levels and reduces inflammation. Lean Protein sources, such as shellfish and white fish are also a good addition to your meals. Yogurt, cheese, eggs, turkey and chicken can be eaten daily or weekly in moderation. Lastly, you should avoid eating processed meats and red meats.

Consume More Veggies and Fruits

On the Mediterranean diet, veggies and Fruits should be the major portion of each meal. The Mediterranean diet recommends the consumption of 7-10 servings of veggies and fruits daily. Come up with creative ways to add more veggies and fruits to your meals, such as eating apple with nut-based butter for a snack, adding cucumber and avocado to your sandwich, and having eggs with added spinach.

Keep Away from Processed Cheese

Eat cheese moderately and avoid processed cheeses. Add an assortment of tasty cheeses to your Mediterranean meals, such as Parmesan or feta in small amounts.

Avoid Using Butter to Cook

The major supply of fat on the Mediterranean diet is olive oil. Trade cooking with butter for heart-healthy fats such as olive oil for improved heart health and lower cholesterol. The type of fat you consume on the Mediterranean diet is very important. Consume poly and monounsaturated fats and hardly any trans fats or saturated fats.

Avoid Refined Grains

Whole grains are known to enhance weight loss, control blood sugar and lower cholesterol. They also contain fiber and vitamin B in high amounts. Trade refined grains such as pasta and white rice for whole grains such as farro, barley and bulgur. Also, legumes and beans have identical health benefits and they can also be consumed as part of your Mediterranean meals.

Choosing your Yogurt

Avoid flavored, high sugar yogurts to avoid falling sick. Add Greek, fermented and plain yogurt to your Mediterranean meals.

Cut Out the Sugar

Sugars, refined flours, crackers and processed cookies should be avoided as much as possible. As a replacement for sugar, fresh fruits such as figs and dates are consumed on the Mediterranean diet.

Eat Nuts as Snack

Nuts contain fiber and protein and also contains poly and monounsaturated fats in high amounts like avocados and olive oil. Some nuts, such as walnuts are loaded with omega-3. What's more, fiber, protein and healthy fats are a flawless match to reduce inflammation, lower cholesterol, stabilize blood sugar and to stay full.

Drink Red Wine Moderately

On the Mediterranean diet, a man should not drink more than 10 ounces in one day, and a woman 5 ounces per day. Don't start drinking, if you don't drink at present.

Mediterranean Pantry Ideas

Whole Grain Ideas

You can pair and blend these whole grains as stir-fries, grain-bowl bases and easy sides. Here are some whole grain ideas for your pantry: brown rice, wheat berries, oats, couscous, barley, farro, buckwheat, bulgur, whole-grain bread.

Veggies and Fruits Ideas

You should shop for your fruit in their season to get the best possible nutrients out of each. Here are some veggies and fruits to keep within reach: peas, peppers, zucchini, onions, beets, Brussels sprouts, cabbage, greens (such as arugula, collards, spinach and kale), artichokes, potatoes, tomatoes, dates, figs, apricots, avocado, grapes, cherries, clementine, pears, oranges, bananas, apples, berries.

Poultry Ideas

On the Mediterranean diet you can eat lean meats in moderate amounts. They should also be eaten infrequently. Lean meats, such as turkey and chicken.

Fish and Seafood Ideas

Fish are the main source of protein on the Mediterranean diet. Here are some fish examples on the diet: Sardines, herring, mackerel, tuna, salmon and other seafood.

Dairy Ideas

Moderate amounts of dairy are okay on the Mediterranean diet. Dairy, such as Greek yogurt, plain yogurt and unprocessed cheeses (such as Parmesan, ricotta, Brie and feta) are acceptable in moderation.

Meat Ideas

Here are some meats loaded with protein, such as lamb, beef and pork. These meats can be eaten occasionally; combined with veggies and whole grains. Eat only a small quantity of lamb per month.

Spices and Herb Ideas

Add this spices and herbs to your meals for the extra flavor. You can use fresh or dry herbs as desired. The following are some herbs and spices that should be within reach: oregano, basil, tarragon, rosemary, sage, mint, garlic, parsley.

Legumes, Seeds and Nut Ideas

You can mix and match for topping your salad, snacks and more. Here are some nuts, seeds and legumes that you can eat on the Mediterranean diet: sesame seeds, pine nuts, cashews, hazelnuts, almonds, walnuts, fava beans and chickpea.

Other Staple Ideas

These staples are also used every now and then on the diet. Keep them at hand: red wine, eggs, canola oil, olive oil.

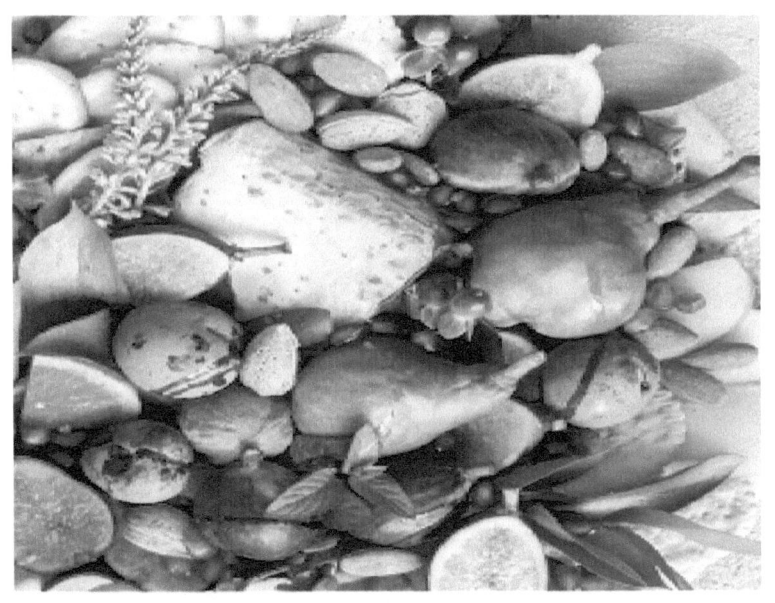

MEDITERRANEAN MEAL GUIDE

Research shows that the Mediterranean diet is comparatively moderate on animal foods and high in healthy plant foods. Nevertheless, enjoying seafood and fish is suggested at least twice weekly. What's more, the Mediterranean diet transcends just eating; it includes enjoying life, sharing meals and regular physical exercise.

What to Eat on the Mediterranean Diet?
Your diet should be filled with foods that are healthy and foods that are not processed.

Healthy Food Options
The following are healthy and whole foods and ingredients that can be eaten on the Mediterranean diet.

Healthy Fats

Avocado oil, avocados, olives, olive oil

Spices and Herbs

Pepper, cinnamon, nutmeg, sage, rosemary, mint, basil, garlic, etc.

Dairy

Greek yogurt, plain yogurt, cheese, etc.

Eggs

Duck eggs, quail eggs, chicken eggs

Poultry

Turkey, duck, chicken

Seafood and Fish

Mussels, crab, clams, oysters, shrimp, mackerel, tuna, trout, sardines, salmon, etc.

Whole Grains

Whole grain bread, whole grain pasta, whole wheat, buckwheat, corn, barley, rye, brown rice, whole oats.

Tubers

Yams, turnips, sweet potatoes, potatoes, etc.

Legumes

Chickpeas, peanuts, pulses, lentils, peas, beans, etc.

Seeds and Nuts

Pumpkin seeds, sunflower seeds, cashews, hazelnuts, macadamia nuts, walnuts, almonds, etc.

Fruits

Peaches, melons, figs, dates, grapes, strawberries, pears, oranges, bananas, apples, etc.

Veggies

Cucumber, Brussels sprouts, carrots, cauliflower, onions, spinach, kale, broccoli, tomatoes, etc.

Healthy Drink Options

Water is the perfect Mediterranean diet beverage. Tea and coffee are also acceptable. Red wine in moderate amounts - about 1 glass each day is okay. Nevertheless, avoid drinking wine if you can't control consumption or you have problems relating to alcoholism. Also, avoid sugar sweetened drinks or drinks that have high sugar amounts.

Here are few snacks options to choose:

Almond butter with apple slices, Greek yogurt, Grapes and berries, Carrots, Fruits, A handful of nuts.

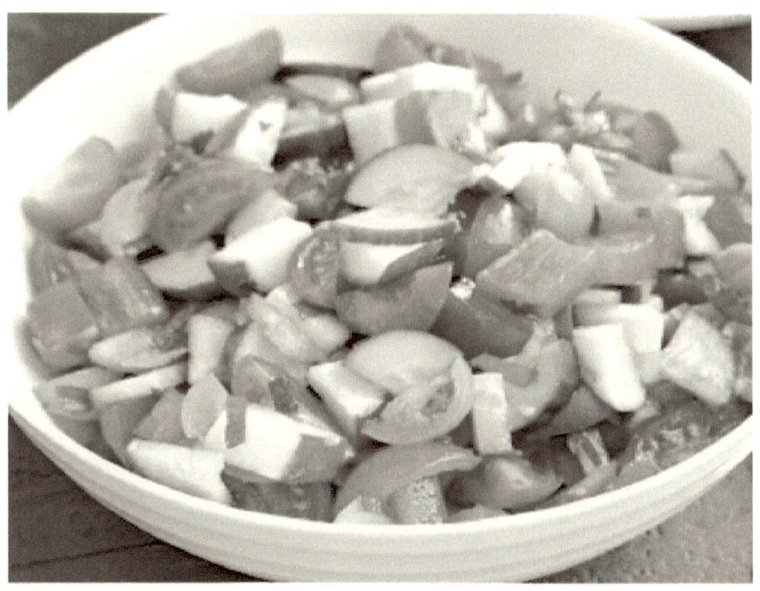

What Not to Eat on the Mediterranean Diet?

Here are some ingredients and foods that are unhealthy and to be avoided:

Highly Processed Foods

Avoid packaged foods that have been processed in a factory. Check food labels well before buying to avoiding stocking up unhealthy and processed foods.

Processed Meat

Processed meats such as hot dogs, processed sausages, etc.

Refined Oils

Refined oils such as cottonseed oil, soybean oil, etc.

Trans Fat

This type of fat is found in several processed foods and margarine.

Refined Grains

Refined wheat pasta, white bread, etc.

Added Sugar

Table sugar, ice cream, candies, soda, etc.

In Summary
Avoid

Highly processed foods, refined oils, refined grains, processed meat, added sugar, and sugar-sweetened drinks and beverages.

Eat Infrequently

Red meat

Eat Moderately

Yogurt, cheese, eggs and poultry

You Can Eat

Olive oil, seafood, fish, spices, herbs, breads, whole grains, potatoes, legumes, seeds, nuts, fruits and veggies.

The Mediterranean is not just a healthy diet, it is a diet that will help you live healthy, love life, and live to the fullest.

30-DAYS MEDITERRANEAN DIET MEAL PLAN

Day One
Breakfast: Barley Raspberry Compote

Lunch: Grilled Turkey Souvlaki

Dinner: Veggie Parmesan Pizza

Snack: Yummy Butter Cookies

Day Two
Breakfast: Cheesy Cilantro Casserole

Lunch: Veggies with Baked Halibut

Dinner: Cheesy Olive Rigatoni Pasta

Snack: Crispy Italian Biscotti

Day Three
Breakfast: Creamy Peaches Baguette

Lunch: Yummy Greek Tzatziki Sauce

Dinner: Rice with Lamb kofta

Snack: Crispy Apple Strudel

Day Four
Breakfast: Mediterranean Apple Galette

Lunch: Turkey Shawarma

Dinner: Greek Roasted Potatoes

Snack: Nutty Grapefruit Cake

Day Five
Breakfast: Greek Yogurt Parfait

Lunch: Olive Feta Pasta

Dinner: Colorful Veggie Bowl with Dressing

Snack: Almond Baklava Rolls

Day Six
Breakfast: Mediterranean Breakfast Donuts

Lunch: Oregano Watermelon Salad

Dinner: Broccoli Panko Salmon

Snack: Cheese Berry Tart

Day Seven
Breakfast: Rich Potato Hash Breakfast + no-sugar coffee with 2 tbsps heavy cream

Lunch: Veggie Tagine + brown rice, couscous or crusty bread

Dinner: Grilled Salmon with Veggie Salsa

Snack: Chocolate Tahini Brownies

Day Eight

Breakfast: Baked Zucchini Omelet with Toast Bread

Lunch: Creamy Mediterranean Hummus + favorite veggies and warm pita

Dinner: Mediterranean Potatoes with Lamb

Snack: Rice Pudding with Pine Nuts

Day Nine

Breakfast: Braised Eggs with Sauce + favorite crusty bread or salad

Lunch: Mediterranean Shrimp Spaghetti

Dinner: Velvety Braised Eggplant

Snack: Rich Shortbread Cookies

Day Ten

Breakfast: Italian Sandwich Breakfast + no-sugar coffee with 2 tbsps heavy cream

Lunch: Veggie Lamb Meatballs with Greens

Dinner: Cheesy Turkey Couscous

Snack: Chocolatey Pistachios Stuffed Dates

Day Eleven

Breakfast: Baked Challah Toast + no-sugar coffee with 2 tbsps heavy cream

Lunch: Creamy Turkey Marsala

Dinner: Turkey Lime Pita Burger

Snack: Yogurt Parfait with Pumpkin

Day Twelve
Breakfast: Spicy Greek Tomato Omelet + crusty bread or salad

Lunch: Arugula Salad with Meatloaf

Dinner: Swiss Chard with Salmon

Snack: Grapefruit Yogurt Crostini

Day Thirteen
Breakfast: East Mediterranean Manakish + olives, (radish, cucumbers, tomato), or feta cheese

Lunch: Cucumber Turkey Salad

Dinner: Basil Turkey Pita

Snack: Nutty Date Bars

Day Fourteen
Breakfast: Carrot Wheat Cake

Lunch: Turkey Zucchini Pizza

Dinner: Mediterranean Lamb Stew + Favorite salad or crusty bread

Snack: Basil Shortbread Cookies

Day Fifteen

Breakfast: Herbs Rich Omelet + a side of Greek olives and favorite bread

Lunch: Feta Tomato Panmolle

Dinner: Pasta with Lebanese Rice

Snack: Peanut Butter Brownies with Pecan

Day Sixteen

Breakfast: Oil Apple Cake

Lunch: Tomato Pasta Salad + crusty bread

Dinner: Lime Scallops with Pasta

Snack: A handful of nuts

Day Seventeen

Breakfast: Mediterranean Tortilla with Salad

Lunch: Turkey Pita Salad

Dinner: Pepper Spinach Gnocchi

Snack: Fruits

Day Eighteen

Breakfast: Rich Fluffy Omelet + warm pita bread and tzatziki sauce

Lunch: Lamb Gremolada

Dinner: Crispy Zucchini Pizza

Snack: Carrots

Day Nineteen

Breakfast: Greek Bread + favorite salad

Lunch: Cheese Tomato Pizza

Dinner: Beans Fish Stew

Snack: Grapes and berries

Day Twenty

Breakfast: Delicious Stuffed Peppers + favorite salad or Greek yogurt

Lunch: Greek Olive Turkey Salad

Dinner: Spicy Skillet Shrimp

Snack: Greek Yogurt

Day Twenty-One

Breakfast: Spinach Feta Frittata

Lunch: Middle Eastern Chicken Burgers

Dinner: Flavored Dijon Turkey

Snack: Almond Butter with Apple Slices

Day Twenty-Two

Breakfast: No-Crust Zucchini Quiche

Lunch: Yummy Greek Scampi

Dinner: Greek Salad + crusty bread

Snack: Carrot

Day Twenty-Three
Breakfast: Poached Fruit Compote

Lunch: Lettuce Wraps with Lamb

Dinner: Rice with Lamb kofta

Snack: Grapefruit Yogurt Crostini

Day Twenty-Four
Breakfast: Nutty Banana Bread

Lunch: Colorful Baked Veggie with Eggs

Dinner: Grilled Salmon with Veggie Salsa

Snack: Rich Shortbread Cookies

Day Twenty-Five
Breakfast: Egg Breakfast Muffins

Lunch: Mediterranean Kofta Kebab + tahini sauce and pita bread

Dinner: Basil Turkey Pita

Snack: Chocolate Tahini Brownies

Day Twenty-Six
Breakfast: Delicious Breakfast Toast

Lunch: Tomato Tuna Steaks

Dinner: Veggie Parmesan Pizza

Snack: Cheesy Grapefruit Cake

Day Twenty-Seven
Breakfast: Rich Potato Hash Breakfast

Lunch: Turkish Beef Meatballs with Pita

Dinner: Swiss Chard with Salmon

Snack: Nutty Grapefruit Cake

Day Twenty-Eight
Breakfast: Creamy Peaches Baguette

Lunch: Feta Turkey Spinach Salad

Dinner: Cheesy Turkey Couscous

Snack: Yummy Butter Cookies

Day Twenty-Nine
Breakfast: Cheesy Cilantro Casserole

Lunch: Cheese Spring Salad

Dinner: Beans Fish Stew

Snack: Crispy Italian Biscotti

Day Thirty

Breakfast: Italian Sandwich Breakfast

Lunch: Bulgur Turkey Salad

Dinner: Lime Scallops with Pasta

Snack: Chocolatey Pistachios Stuffed Dates

BREAKFAST

Delicious Breakfast Toast

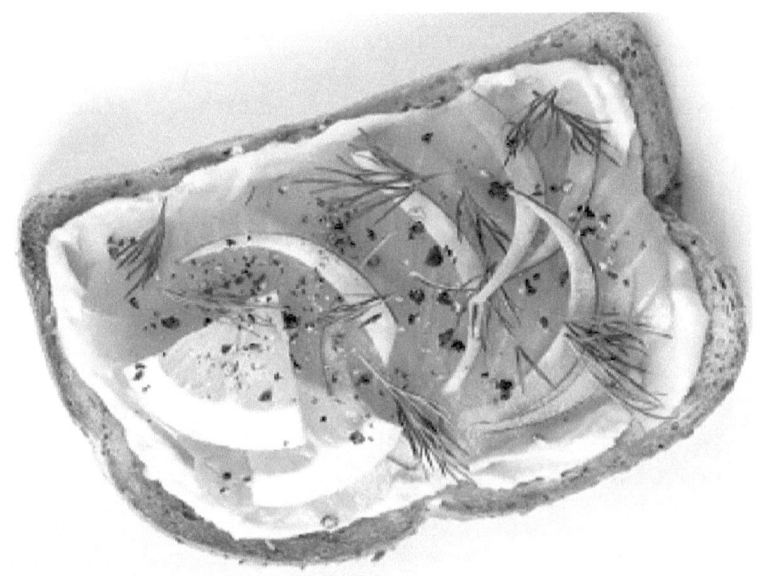

Preparation Time: 10 minutes

Cook Time: 0 minutes

Serves: 4 servings

Ingredients

1/2 cup store-bought hummus

4 (toasted) thick whole wheat or whole grain bread slices

1 handful baby arugula

Harissa, to taste

1-2 (sliced into rounds) Roma tomatoes

1 (sliced into rounds) cucumber

Feta cheese, crumbled

2 tablespoons kalamata olives, chopped

Preparation

1. Add 2 tablespoons hummus on each bread slice and top with harissa.

2. Add every other topping and arugula on each bread slice.

3. Serve and enjoy.

Nutritional Information/Serving

Calories 166 kcal, Protein 6.1g, Total Carbs 29.4g, Sodium 97.6mg, Total Fat 4.2g

Egg Breakfast Muffins

Preparation Time: 15 minutes

Cook Time: 25 minutes

Serves: 12 servings

Ingredients

1 (chopped) small red bell pepper

Olive oil

1 (chopped finely) shallot

12 halved cherry tomatoes

3-4 ounces boneless (cooked & shredded) turkey

6-10 (pitted and chopped) kalamata olives

1 handful crumbled feta

1/2 cup fresh chopped cilantro

Salt and Pepper

8 large eggs

1/2 teaspoon Spanish paprika

Preparation

1. Set a rack in the middle of your oven and heat up oven to 350°F.

2. Prepare a greased 12-cup muffin tin with olive oil.

3. Add crumbled feta, cilantro, turkey, olives, shallots, tomatoes and peppers into a bowl and combine.

4. Split feta mixture into the prepared muffin tin, until two third of the way full.

5. Add spices, pepper, salt and eggs into a big bowl and whisk until combined.

6. Top feta mixture with the egg mixture.

Note: Leave enough room at the top of each muffin cup.

7. Transfer muffin pan into the center rack of the oven and bake until eggs are ready, for about 25 minutes.

8. Let sit to cool and loosen muffins around the edges with a sharp knife.

9. Serve and enjoy.

Nutritional Information/Serving

Calories 67 kcal, Protein 4.6g, Total Carbs 1.2g, Sodium 161.4mg, Total Fat 4.7g

Nutty Banana Bread

Preparation Time: 15 minutes

Cook Time: 55 minutes

Serves: 14 slices

Ingredients

1/2 cup organic honey

1/3 cup olive oil

2 mashed bananas, ripe

2 eggs

1/4 cup milk, low-fat

2 tablespoons plain yogurt, no-fat

1 teaspoon vanilla extract

1 teaspoon baking soda

1/2 teaspoon cinnamon, ground

1/2-3/4 teaspoon cardamom, ground

1 1/3 cup wheat flour

1/2 teaspoon nutmeg, ground

1/3 cup walnut hearts, chopped

6 (pitted and chopped) dates

Preparation

1. Heat up oven to 325°F.

2. Add honey and olive oil into a big bowl and whisk until combined.

3. Add eggs into the honey mixture and whisk until combined.

4. Add nutmeg, cinnamon, cardamom, vanilla extract, baking soda, milk, yogurt and banana into the honey mixture and whisk until combined.

5. Stir in the wheat flour using a spatula.

6. Add walnuts and dates into the batter and stir until evenly distributed and combined.

7. Prepare 5 3/4-by-3" lightly oiled nonstick loaf pan.

8. Empty the batter into the prepared pan and shake pan lightly until batter is spread evenly.

9. Transfer loaf pan into the preheated oven and bake until an inserted toothpick comes out clean for 55 minutes.

10. Take out bread from the oven and let sit for 10 minutes until cooled.

11. Move bread to wire rack for about 20 minutes until cool.

12. Slice bread, serve and enjoy.

Nutritional Information/Serving

Calories 172 kcal, Protein 2.4g, Total Carbs 28.8g, Sodium 104.1mg, Total Fat 5.9g

Poached Fruit Compote

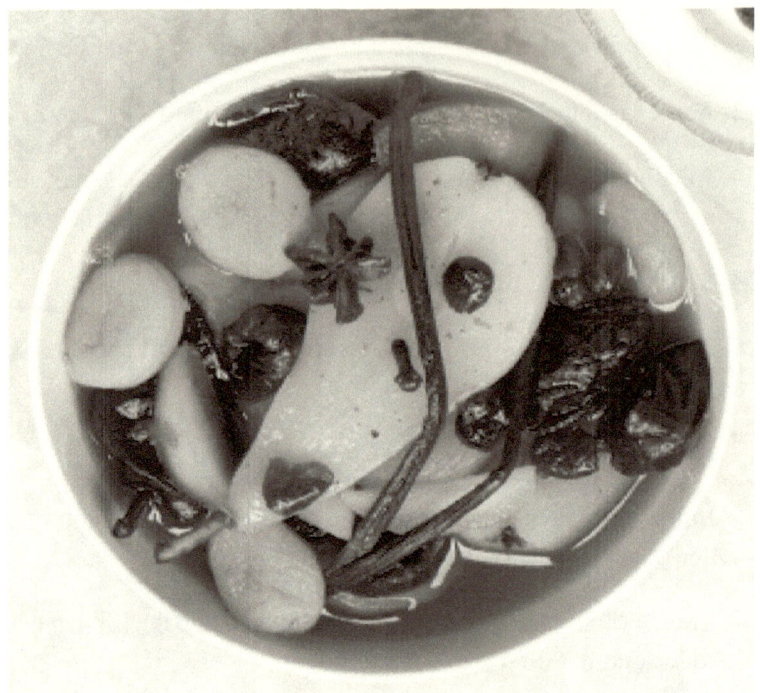

Preparation Time: 15 minutes

Cook Time: 5 minutes

Serves: 10 servings

Ingredients

1 pound (pitted and halved) cherries

3-4 (halved, pitted and sliced thin) peaches

2 cups red wine

1 teaspoon cinnamon, ground

1 1/2 cup Greek yogurt, plain no-free

3/4 cup cane sugar

Honey

1 teaspoon vanilla extract

Preparation

1. Add cherries and peaches into a big bowl.

2. Shake cinnamon over peaches, toss to combine and let sit until needed.

3. Add sugar and wine into a saucepan over high.

4. Heat until sugar is fully dissolved, for 5 minutes.

5. Empty sugar syrup over the cherries, place lid over bowl and let sit until cooled for 1 hour.

6. Get rid of the syrup, retaining just a small cup for later use.

7. Add honey, vanilla extract and Greek yogurt into a small bowl and combine.

8. Serve fruit compote, topped with a blob of Greek yogurt mixture and a little poaching syrup.

Nutritional Information/Serving

Calories 167 kcal, Total Carbs 10.9g, Sodium 14.6mg, Total Fat 0g

No-Crust Zucchini Quiche

Preparation Time: 10 minutes

Cook Time: 35 minutes

Serves: 8 slices

Ingredients

Olive oil

1 (sliced thinly into rounds) tomato, medium

3 (sliced into rounds) shallots

1 (slice into rounds) zucchini

1 teaspoon (divided) sweet paprika

Salt and pepper

2 tablespoons Parmesan, grated

1/2 cup shredded mozzarella, part-skim

2/3 cup skim milk

3 (beaten) eggs, large

1/2 cup (sifted) white whole wheat flour

1/4 teaspoon baking powder

1/4 cup packed fresh cilantro

Preparation

1. Heat up oven to 350ºF.

2. Add the tomato slices onto paper towel, arrange and season evenly with salt.

3. Let tomato slices sit for some minutes and pat dry.

4. In the meantime, add 2 tablespoons olive oil into a big skillet over med-heat.

5. Heat oil until shimmering.

Note: don't over heat, oil should not be smoky.

6. Add shallots and zucchini into the hot oil and season 1/2 teaspoon sweet paprika, pepper and salt.

7. Increase heat a little and saute the zucchini mixture until finely colored and softened; toss often.

Note: Zucchini will have some brown spots.

8. Lightly oil the base of a 9" pie dish.

9. Transfer the cooked veggies into the prepared dish.

10. Add the tomato slices over the zucchini mixture and arrange.

11. Spread Parmesan and mozzarella cheese over mixture evenly.

12. Add fresh cilantro, flour, baking powder, 1/2 teaspoon paprika, milk and eggs into a bowl and whisk until combined.

13. Empty the egg mixture into the dish.

14. Transfer pie dish into the preheated oven and bake until egg mixture is hardened, for about 30 minutes.

15. Take out quiche from the oven, let sit to cool before you serve.

16. Serve and enjoy.

Nutritional Information/Serving

Calories 145 kcal, Protein 8.4g, Total Carbs 16.5g, Sodium 252.2mg, Total Fat 5.6g

Spinach Feta Frittata

Preparation Time: 10 minutes

Cook Time: 12 minutes

Serves: 8 slices

Ingredients

1/4 cup milk

8 eggs

1/2 teaspoon dill weed

1 teaspoon basil, dried

1/2 teaspoon paprika

1/2 teaspoon black pepper

6 ounces (thawed and squeeze out water completely) chopped spinach, frozen

1 pinch salt

1 cup fresh chopped cilantro

1/2 cup yellow onion, chopped finely

3 minced garlic cloves

3 tablespoons fresh mint leaves, chopped

Olive oil

3-4 ounces feta cheese, crumbled

Preparation

1. Heat up oven to 375°F.

2. Add 1 pinch salt, spices and eggs into a big bowl and whisk until combined.

3. Add every other ingredient with the spinach into the egg mixture and stir until well combined.

4. Add 2 tablespoons olive oil into a 12" cast iron skillet and heat until it shimmers.

Note: don't over heat, oil should not be smoky.

5. Empty the spinach egg mixture into the heated oil, spread mixture by shaking lightly.

6. Adjust heat to med-high and cook until eggs are set for about 4 minutes.

7. Move cast iron skillet into the preheated oven and bake until eggs are set and well cooked, for 8 minutes.

8. Serve with Mediterranean Salad.

Nutritional Information/Serving

Calories 152 kcal, Protein 9.8g, Total Carbs 4.9g, Sodium 347.7mg, Total Fat 10.7g

Delicious Stuffed Peppers

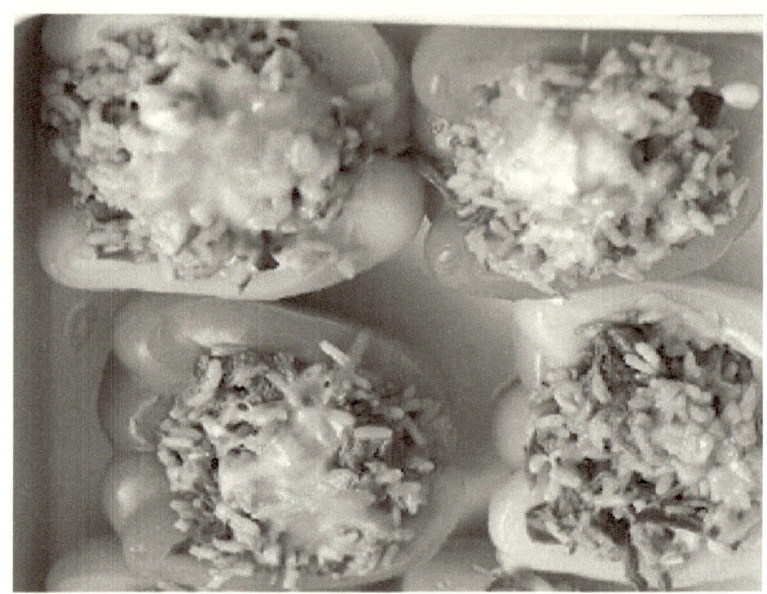

Preparation Time: 10 minutes

Cook Time: 15 minutes

Serves: 6 servings

Ingredients

Water

3 (halve lengthways and remove core) bell peppers

6 ounces (sliced and chopped) mushrooms

Olive oil

10-12 ounces (peeled and diced small) gold potatoes

1 cup yellow onion, chopped

3/4 teaspoon hot paprika

Salt and pepper, to taste

3/4 teaspoon cumin, organic

3/4 teaspoon coriander, organic

3 chopped garlic cloves

1/2 teaspoon turmeric, organic

1/2 cup packed fresh chopped cilantro

1/2 cup cherry tomatoes, chopped

6 eggs

Preparation

1. Heat up oven to 350°F.

2. Place pepper boats on a baking dish with the cut side up.

3. Add 1 cup water into the bottom of the baking dish.

4. Place aluminum foil over baking dish until covered.

5. Transfer baking dish into the preheated oven and bake for 10-15 minutes.

6. In the meantime, add mushrooms into a 12" cast iron skillet over high heat.

7. Stir cook often until finely browned.

8. Sprinkle salt over mushrooms and remove mushrooms into a plate and let sit until needed.

9. Adjust heat to med-high.

10. Add 2 tablespoons olive oil into the skillet until it shimmers.

11. Add potatoes and onions into the hot oil and sprinkle with the spices, pepper and salt.

12. Stir cook potato mixture for 5 minutes.

13. Add garlic into the potato mixture and stir cook for 5-7 more minutes until potatoes are softened.

14. Add cilantro, tomatoes and cooked mushrooms into the potato mixture and stir until combined before removing from heat.

15. Take out pepper boats from the baking dish and reserve the cooking water.

16. Add potato filling into the pepper boats until filled - 3/4 of the way.

17. Crack an egg over potato filling into each pepper boat.

18. Tent aluminum foil over baking dish, transfer into the preheated oven and bake until eggs are just-set for 18-20 minutes.

19. Serve and enjoy.

Nutritional Information/Serving

Calories 179 kcal, Protein 9.5g, Total Carbs 15.6g, Sodium 94.3mg, Total Fat 9.1g

Greek Bread

Preparation Time: 30 minutes

Cook Time: 45 minutes

Serves: 16 slices

Ingredients

5 1/2 cups flour, all-purpose

2 1/4 teaspoons active dry yeast

1 1/3 cup milk

1/2 cup sugar

1 teaspoon fine salt

5 tablespoons butter, unsalted

Egg wash = 1 teaspoon water + 1 beaten egg

2 (beaten) large eggs

1/4 teaspoon vanilla extract

2 tablespoons anise seed

Olive oil

3 (dyed red and dried fully) hard-boiled eggs

2-4 tablespoons sesame seeds, toasted

Preparation

1. Add 1 tablespoon sugar, 1 tablespoon flour, yeast and 1/3 cup hot water into a bowl, combine and pour into a stand mixer bowl and whisk lightly.

2. Place towel over mixer until covered and let sit until bubbly for 10 minutes.

3. Add milk into a small saucepan and heat for about 4-6 minutes until milk edges are bubbly.

4. Remove saucepan from heat, add salt, remaining sugar and butter into the milk and stir until wholly incorporated.

5. Let mixture sit until cooled, for 5 minutes.

6. Add milk mixture into the flour mixture and stir until wholly incorporated using the mixer's paddle attachment.

7. Add the 2 beaten eggs into the batter while the paddle runs.

8. Slowly vanilla extract and anise seed into the batter and beat until combined and soft dough is formed.

9. Adjust paddle speed to med-high until dough is released from the bowl sides.

10. Lightly flour a flat work surface and add the dough.

11. Knead dough for about 5 minutes until a smooth consistency is reached.

12. Oil a bowl lightly and add the kneaded dough.

13. Place lid over bowl until covered, put covered bowl in a closed warm are until dough rises, for about 1 hour 30 minutes.

14. Hit dough until flattened and moved to the floured flat surface.

15. Slice dough in 3 even sections and roll into a 16" rope.

16. Transfer dough ropes into a big parchment paper lined baking sheet.

17. Press the ropes at an end and knit loosely.

18. Form dough weaves into a ring and press on the other side.

19. Expand dough circle, about 3 1/2" wide hole in the middle and 10" diagonally.

20. Place a clean towel over dough and return into the warm area for an hour until it rises.

21. Brush olive oil over dyed eggs and clean with a paper towel.

22. Softly add the dyed eggs into 3 equidistant points on the dough, cover and place back in the warm area.

23. Let dough sit until doubled, for 1 hour extra.

24. Heat up oven to 350°F.

25. Brush dough with egg wash until evenly covered and top evenly with toasted sesame seeds.

26. Transfer into the preheated oven and bake knitted dough until a fine deep golden brown is reached, for about 45 minutes.

Note: check for doneness by tapping to hear if a hallow sound comes back.

27. Let sit for 30 minutes until cool before you serve.

28. Serve as desired.

Nutritional Information/Serving

Calories 252 kcal, Protein 7.3g, Total Carbs 40.6g, Sodium 175.8mg, Total Fat 6.6g

Rich Fluffy Omelet

Preparation Time: 5 minutes

Cook Time: 2 minutes

Serves: 2 servings

Ingredients

2 tablespoons milk, no-fat

4 eggs, large

1/4 teaspoon allspice, ground

1/2 teaspoon Spanish paprika

1/2 teaspoon pepper

1/2 teaspoon salt

1 1/2 teaspoon virgin olive oil

Top with

2 tablespoons (pitted and sliced) Kalamata olives

1/2 cup (halved) cherry tomatoes

2 tablespoons fresh chopped cilantro

1/4-1/3 cup (drained and quartered) artichoke hearts, marinated

2 tablespoons fresh chopped mint

Preparation

1. Add pepper, salt, spices, milk and eggs into a bowl and whisk forcefully and swiftly until combined.

2. Add olive oil into a 10" nonstick skillet and heat until the oil shimmers.

3. Toss skillet lightly until the base is evenly coated with oil.

4. Add egg mixture into the oiled skillet and stir with a wooden spoon for 5 seconds.

5. Moved the cooked part of the egg to the middle of the pan and tilt skillet to allow uncooked egg to move to the edges.

6. Cook until egg bottom is just golden for a minute and the egg is just set.

7. Take pan off heat, and add the toppings to the middle of the omelet.

8. Fold omelet and top again with any remaining ingredient.

9. Sprinkle any remaining herb over folded omelet and slice in two.

10. Serve at once, as desired and enjoy.

Nutritional Information/Serving

Calories 167 kcal, Protein 13.8g, Total Carbs 3.7g, Sodium 771.2mg, Total Fat 10.7g

Mediterranean Tortilla with Salad

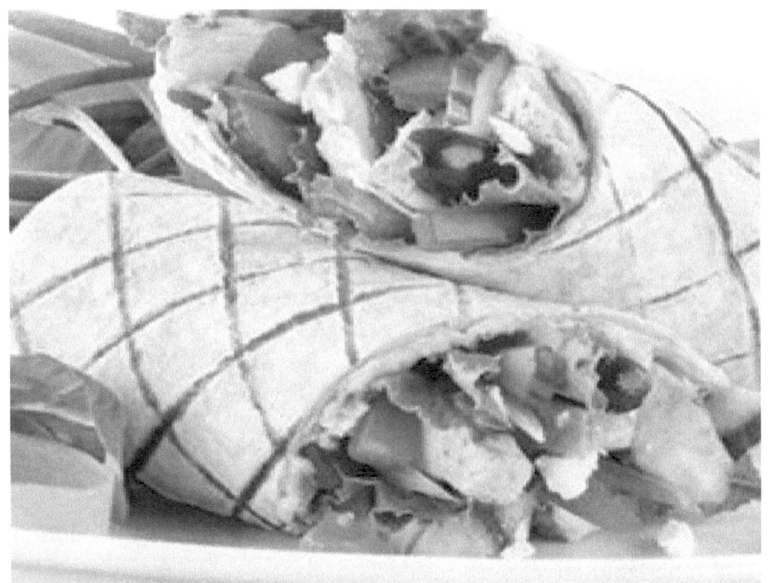

Preparation Time: 15 minutes

Cook Time: 30 minutes

Serves: 6 servings

Ingredients

Salt

10 eggs, medium

1 teaspoon basil, dried

1 teaspoon sweet Spanish paprika

1 1/2 pounds (peeled, halved and sliced crossways) russet potatoes

1 cup olive oil

4 (trim and chop both green and white parts) scallions

1 (peeled, halved and sliced crossways) yellow onion, large

Salad

8 ounces baby arugula

8 ounces baby spinach

1 teaspoon lemon pepper seasoning

Salt and pepper, to taste

Olive oil

1–2 teaspoon lime juice

Preparation

1. Add basil, paprika, salt and eggs into a big bowl, whisk until combined and let sit until needed.

2. Prepare a 10" nonstick oven-proof skillet.

3. Add olive oil into the skillet over med-high heat.

4. Heat oil until it shimmers and add the scallions, onions and potatoes into the heated skillet.

5. Adjust heat to med-low and stir cook until potatoes are softened, for 25 minutes.

6. Heat up oven to 400°F.

7. Drain and reserve oil until needed and sprinkle salt over softened potatoes.

8. Whisk eggs again and add the potato mixture.

9. Add 3 tablespoon of the used olive oil into a skillet over med-heat.

10. Heat olive oil, add the potato/egg mixture into the skillet with oil and press lightly until the top becomes even.

11. Adjust heat to med-low.

12. Cook potato/egg mixture for 2 minutes and move mixture with the skillet into the preheated oven.

13. Bake mixture for 5 minutes until well cooked and flip onto a platter, garnished with chopped scallions.

14. Let sit to cool for 10 minutes before you serve.

15. In the meantime, add every salad ingredient into a bowl and toss until combined.

16. Serve tortillas with salad and enjoy.

Nutritional Information/Serving

Calories 381, Protein 13.3g, Total Carbs 24g, Sodium 513.3mg, Total Fat 26.7g

Oil Apple Cake

Preparation Time: 20 minutes

Cook Time: 45 minutes

Serves: 12 servings

Ingredients

Orange, juiced

2 (peeled and finely chopped) fuji apples, large

1/2 teaspoon cinnamon, ground

3 cups flour, all-purpose

1 teaspoon baking powder

1/2 teaspoon nutmeg, ground

1 cup sugar

1 teaspoon baking soda

2 eggs, large

1 cup olive oil

2/3 cup (soak for 15 minutes in warm water and drain well) gold raisins

Dust with

Powdered sugar

Preparation

1. Heat up oven to 350°F.

2. Add just enough orange juice to cover and the apple chunks into a bowl and toss until wholly coated.

3. Sift the flour, baking soda, baking powder, nutmeg and cinnamon together in a big bowl and let sit until needed.

4. Fit a whisk to a stand mixer and add olive oil and sugar into the stand mixer bowl.

5. Mix to combine for 2 minutes on low speed.

6. Add an egg per time into the running mixer and keep mixing until the mixture is multiplied in size, runny and thicker, for about 2 minutes.

7. Repeat process with the remaining egg.

8. Make a hole in the center of the cinnamon/flour mixture and add the egg/olive oil mixture.

9. Stir wet and dry mixture until combined and a thick batter is formed using a wooden spoon

10. Get rid of citrus juice from the soaked apples and wholly drain the raisins.

11. Add apples and drained raisins into the batter and stir until evenly incorporated.

12. Prepare a parchment paper lined 9" cake pan.

13. Scoop batter into the prepared pan and spread at the top until even with the back end of your spoon.

Note: batter should remain thick.

14. Transfer cake pan into the preheated oven and bake cake until an inserted toothpick comes out clean, for 45 minutes.

15. Let sit until wholly cool, remove cake with the parchment paper and place on a platter.

16. Sprinkle powdered sugar over cake.

Nutritional Information/Serving

Calories 294 kcal, Protein 5.3g, Total Carbs 47.7g, Total Fat 11g

Herbs Rich Omelet

Preparation Time: 20 minutes

Cook Time: 20 minutes

Serves: 6 servings

Ingredients

2 cups parsley leaves, flat-leaf

5 tablespoons olive oil

1 cup fresh dill, coarsely chopped

2 cups cilantro, tender stems and leaves

1 1/2 teaspoons baking powder

6 (trim and chop roughly) scallions

3/4 teaspoon green cardamom, ground

1 teaspoon kosher salt

1/2 teaspoon cumin, ground

3/4 teaspoon cinnamon, ground

6 eggs, large

1/4 teaspoon black pepper, ground

Preparation

1. Heat up an oven with a rack in the top-center position to 375ºF.

2. Fit the base of a 9" round cake pan with parchment paper and generously oil the cake pan inside until wholly coated with 2 tablespoons olive oil.

Tip: coat the parchment paper at the base on the two sides.

3. Add 3 tablespoons olive, scallions, dill, cilantro and parsley into a food processor and process until desired consistency is reached and let sit until needed.

4. Add pepper, cumin, cinnamon, cardamom, salt and baking powder into a big bowl and whisk to combine.

5. Add 2 eggs into the baking powder mixture and whisk until combined.

6. Whisk in the remaining 4 eggs until just combined.

7. Fold in the processed parsley mixture into the eggs until incorporated.

8. Empty egg mixture into the prepared pan and transfer into the preheated oven.

9. Bake egg mixture for about 20-25 minutes until the middle of the egg is solid.

10. Let sit for 10 minutes to cool before loosening with a knife round the edges of pan.

11. Slice omelet into wedges and serve warm.

Nutritional Information/Serving

Calories 183 kcal, Protein 7.1g, Total Carbs 2.7g, Total Fat 16.7g

Carrot Wheat Cake

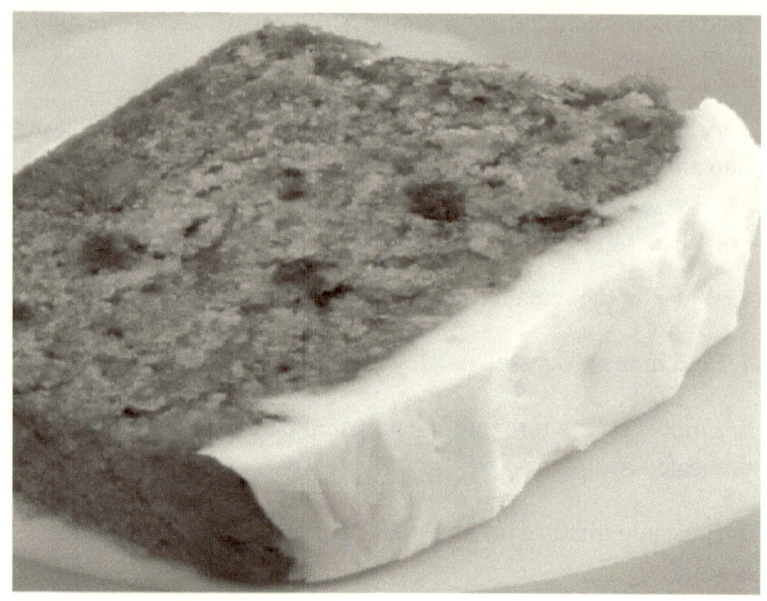

Preparation Time: 10 minutes

Cook Time: 60 minutes

Serves: 12 servings

Ingredients

1/2 cup low-fat Greek yogurt

1/2 cup olive oil

1/2 cup honey, dark

1/3 cup low-fat 2% milk

2 1/4 cup whole wheat flour

3 (room temp) eggs

1/2 teaspoon salt

1 1/2 teaspoons baking powder

1/2 teaspoon cardamom, ground

4 teaspoons cinnamon, ground

2 cups carrots, finely grated

1/4 teaspoon ginger, ground

1/3 cup walnuts, chopped

6 (pitted and chopped finely) Medjool dates

Dust with

Sugar, powdered

Preparation

1. Heat up oven to 350°F.

2. Add milk, Greek yogurt and olive oil into a big bowl and whisk until combined.

3. Add an egg at a time and keep whisking until fully incorporated. Repeat process until no egg remains.

4. Add spices, salt, baking powder and wheat flour into a second bowl and whisk to combine.

5. Use a wooden spatula to slowly add and mix in the flour mixture into the egg mixture until combined.

6. Fold in the grated carrots into the batter until mixed, add the walnuts and dates until fully incorporated.

Tip: mix well with the wooden spoon.

7. Prepare a parchment paper lined 9" square baking dish and add the batter.

8. Transfer cake pan into the preheated oven and bake until an inserted toothpick comes out clean, for an hour.

9. Let cake sit until cooled.

10. Dust with powdered sugar and slice into 12 slices.

Nutritional Information/Serving

Calories 167 kcal, Protein 5g, Total Carbs 20.2g, Sodium 138.1mg, Total Fat 8.6g

East Mediterranean Manakish

Preparation Time: 30 minutes

Cook Time: 8 minutes

Serves: 8 servings

Ingredients (dough)

1/2 teaspoon sugar

1 cup water, lukewarm

3 cups all-purpose flour, unbleached

2 1/4 teaspoons active dry yeast

2 tablespoons olive oil

1 teaspoon salt

Top with

1/2 cup olive oil

7-8 tablespoons Za'atar spice

Preparation

1. Add yeast, sugar and water into a small bowl, combine and let sit to foam for 10 minutes.

2. Add olive salt and flour into a big bowl and combine.

3. Use clean hands to work the flour mixture.

4. Make a hole in the middle of the flour mixture and add the water mixture.

5. Stir water and flour mixture until a tender dough consistency is formed.

6. Lightly flour a flat work surface and add the dough.

7. Knead dough until dough is smooth, elastic and dough lose stickiness, and form into a ball.

8. Oil a mixing bowl lightly.

9. Transfer dough ball into the prepared bowl, place a damp cloth over bowl until covered and store in a warm area until the dough rises, for 1 1/2 hour.

10. Hit dough until flattened and knead for a short while before forming into 8 smaller balls.

11. Return dough balls onto the floured flat surface, cover again and let sit for 30 more minutes until risen.

12. In the meantime, add olive oil and za'atar spice into a bowl and combine.

13. Heat up oven to 400°F.

14. Transfer a big baking sheet into the preheated oven.

15. Oil the heated baking sheet lightly and let sit.

16. Press each dough ball into 5" wide rounds and make a well at the center.

17. Add 1 tablespoon of the za'atar mixture in each well and transfer the topped dough rounds into the prepared baking dish.

Note: do not over crowd the baking sheet.

18. Transfer baking sheet into the preheated oven and bake until dough is just browned at the edges and the base.

19. Take out manakish from the oven and let sit until za'atar topping settles in and dries out.

20. Serve warm with desired servings.

Nutritional Information/Serving

Calories 306 kcal, Protein 5.5g, Total Carbs 38.2g, Total Fat 14.7g

Spicy Greek Tomato Omelet

Preparation Time: 5 minutes

Cook Time: 15 minutes

Serves: 4 servings

Ingredients

1 (sliced into 4 thick slices) tomato, large

Olive oil

2 tablespoons Greek feta cheese, crumbled

1 minced garlic clove

1 tablespoon fresh mint leaves, chopped

7 eggs, large

1/2 teaspoon sweet paprika

1/2 teaspoon baking powder

1/2 teaspoon coriander

1/2 teaspoon dill weed

Salt and black pepper, to taste

Preparation

1. Add olive oil into an oven-secure nonstick skillet over med-heat.

2. Spread sliced tomatoes into the skillet in a single layer.

3. Sprinkle minced garlic over tomato layer and cook without stirring for about 5 minutes until tomatoes are a little dry and tenderized.

4. Add feta cheese into the tomato mixture and cook until slightly melted.

5. In the meantime, add eggs into a big bowl, add pepper, salt, spices, fresh mint and baking powder and whisk to combine.

6. Adjust heat to med-high heat.

7. Empty egg mixture into the skillet over the tomato mixture.

8. Place lid loosely over skillet and cook until egg tops are just hardened.

9. Transfer skillet to oven and broil for a short time until egg is fully cooked.

Note: watch eggs to avoid burning.

10. Serve as desired.

Nutritional Information/Serving

Calories 179 kcal, Protein 11.8g, Total Carbs 3.4g, Sodium 208.1mg, Total Fat 13g

Baked Challah Toast

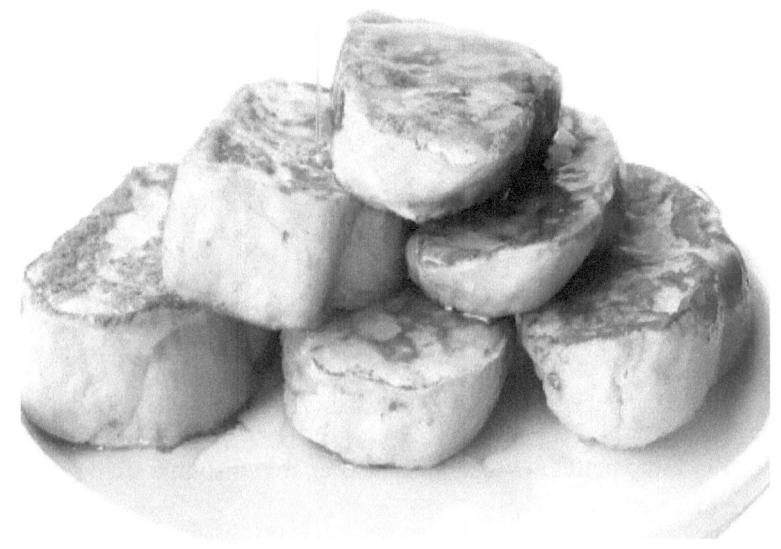

Preparation Time: 15 minutes

Cook Time: 30 minutes

Serves: 6 servings

Ingredients

1 tablespoon cold butter, unsalted + 2 tablespoons soft butter, unsalted

6–8 (3/4" thick) challah bread slices

2 eggs, large

1 cup plain yogurt, reduced-fat

2 teaspoons vanilla extract

1 tablespoon honey

1/4 cup milk, reduced-fat

Honey Syrup

1 cup water

1 cup honey

1/4 teaspoon lemon juice

Dust with

Powdered sugar

Preparation

1. Prepare a big 10-by-14" baking dish.

2. Butter bread slices on one side with 1 tablespoon soft butter.

3. Place the buttered bread into the prepared dish in a single layer with the buttered-side down.

4. Fill any remaining space with bread pieces until covered with the buttered side down.

Note: every crevice and corner should be filled with buttered bread.

5. Add vanilla, honey, eggs and yogurt into a big bowl and whisk until combined.

6. Pour yogurt mixture into the baking dish over the bread and use a spatula to spread until bread is evenly covered.

Tip: Pull few bread slices to allow yogurt mixture soak in.

7. Place lid over baking dish and transfer into a refrigerator for 8 hours or overnight.

8. When ready to cook, heat up oven to 350°F.

9. Set rack in the top-center position of the oven.

10. Spot cold butter throughout challah and top with 1/4 cup of milk until evenly covered.

11. Transfer baking dish into the preheated oven and bake until challah is almost solid when touch and yogurt mixture is hardened.

12. Broil challah until golden brown on the top for 2 minutes.

Note: be careful not to burn.

13. In the meantime, add water and honey into a small saucepan over med-high heat, combine and bring to boiling, stirring every now and then.

14. Adjust heat to simmering and simmer for 20 minutes or so.

15. Take saucepan off heat and let sit until just cooled.

16. Add lemon juice and stir until wholly incorporated.

17. Sprinkle powdered sugar over baked challah toast and top with preferred fruit.

18. Serve baked challah with honey syrup. Enjoy.

Nutritional Information/Serving

Calories 452 kcal, Protein 10.8g, Total Carbs 82.1g, Sodium 62mg, Total Fat 10.7g

Italian Sandwich Breakfast

Preparation Time: 10 minutes

Cook Time: 4 minutes

Serves: 4 servings

Ingredients

2 tablespoons olive oil

1 cup ricotta cheese, part-skim

Salt and pepper, to taste

1/2 teaspoon dried thyme

4–8 fresh basil leaves

4 slices toasted Italian bread

3 (sliced thin) radishes

1 sliced Roma tomato

4 prosciutto slices

2 tablespoons (drained) roasted red pepper in oil

1 tablespoon shelled pistachios, crushed

4 eggs, poached

Preparation

1. Add ricotta cheese into a small bowl, add the pepper, salt, dried thyme and olive oil and use a fork to beat until combined.

2. Cover each toasted bread slice with the cheese mixture.

3. Add every other ingredient on the cheese mixture over each slice of bread.

4. Serve and enjoy.

Nutritional Information/Serving

Calories 439 kcal, Protein 20.4g, Total Carbs 35.5g, Sodium 460.7mg, Total Fat 22.2g

Braised Eggs with Sauce

Preparation Time: 10 minutes

Cook Time: 20 minutes

Serves: 6 servings

Ingredients

1 chopped yellow onion, large

Olive oil

2 (peel and chop) garlic cloves

2 chopped green peppers

1 teaspoon sweet paprika

1 teaspoon coriander, ground

Salt and pepper, to taste

1/2 teaspoon ground cumin

1/2 cup tomato sauce

6 (chopped) tomatoes, chopped

6 eggs, large

1 teaspoon sugar

1/4 cup fresh chopped mint leaves

1/4 cup fresh chopped cilantro

Preparation

1. Add 3 tablespoons olive oil into a big cast iron skillet and heat.

2. Add pepper, salt, spices, garlic, green peppers and onions into the heated oil and stir cook for about 10 minutes until veggies are softened.

3. Add sugar, tomato sauce and the tomatoes into the skillet and simmer for about 10-12 minutes until the mixture reduces.

4. Check for seasoning and adjust as desired.

5. Make six wells in the mixture with a wooden spoon.

6. Crack an egg into each well, adjust heat to low, place lid over skillet and cook until egg whites are hardened.

7. Remove cover, add extra black pepper as desired, add mint and fresh chopped cilantro.

8. Serve as desired wit crusty bread or warm pita.

Nutritional Information/Serving

Calories 154 kcal, Protein 9g, Total Carbs 14.1g, Sodium 86.3mg, Total Fat 7.8g

Baked Zucchini Omelet with Toast Bread

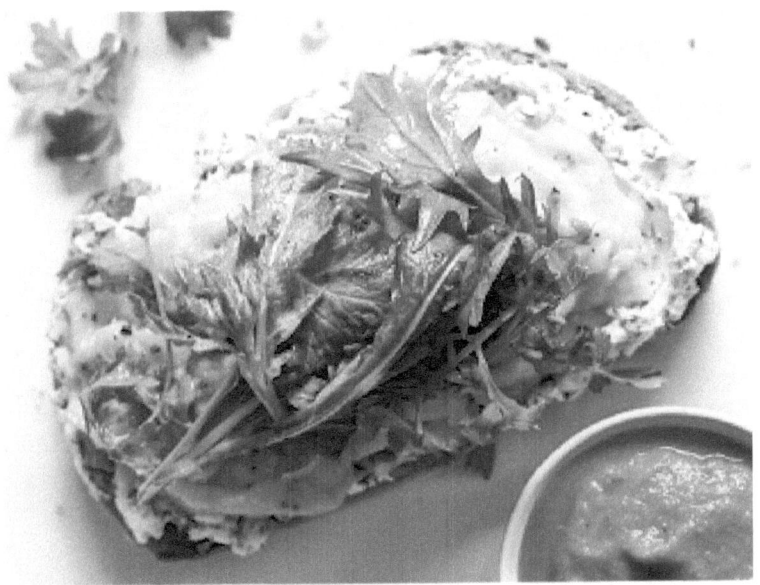

Preparation Time: 10 minutes

Cook Time: 20 minutes

Serves: 6 servings

Ingredients

Salt

2 (sliced into thin rounds) zucchini

1 (sliced thin) small onion

2 tablespoons olive oil

30 (remove stems and tear leaves) fresh mint leaves

1/2 teaspoon garlic powder

1 pinch red pepper flakes

8 eggs, large

2 (remove crust and soak in 1/3 cup milk) toasted bread slices

1/2 teaspoon baking powder

Serve with

Tomato slices

Lime juice

Preparation

1. Heat up oven to 350°F.

2. Sprinkle a small amount of salt over slices of zucchini, let sit for 15 minutes and pat dry.

3. Add olive oil into a 10" cast iron skillet over med-heat.

4. Add onions and zucchini into the heated oil and cook over med-high heat until veggies are golden and softened, for 5-7 minutes.

5. Add 3/4 of the mint leaves and reserve the remaining.

6. Remove skillet from heat and let zucchini mixture sit to cool.

7. Add baking powder, crushed red pepper, salt and eggs into an average bowl and whisk to combine.

8. Drain off excess milk from bread slices by squeezing and then, break bread slices apart with clean hands.

9. Add bread pieces into the egg mixture and lightly whisk until combined.

10. Add onions and zucchini mixture into the egg mixture and stir until wholly incorporated.

11. Add a small amount of olive oil into the same skillet.

12. Empty bread/egg mixture into the skillet and transfer into the preheated oven.

13. Bake until omelet looks well-cooked at the top, for 15-20 minutes.

14. Serve with tomato slices and lime juice, and garnish with the reserved torn mint leaves.

Nutritional Information/Serving

Calories 208 kcal, Protein 11.6g, Total Carbs 13.4g, Sodium 535.6mg, Total Fat 12.8g

Rich Potato Hash Breakfast

Preparation Time: 10 minutes

Cook Time: 14 minutes

Serves: 4 servings

Ingredients

1 (chopped) yellow onion, small

Olive oil

2 (diced) russet potatoes

2 (chopped) garlic cloves

1 cup (drained and rinsed) canned chickpeas

Salt and pepper, to taste

1 1/2 teaspoons allspice, ground

1 pound (remove hard ends and chop into 1/4" pieces) baby asparagus

1 teaspoon basil, dried

1 teaspoon Za'atar

1 teaspoon coriander

1 teaspoon sweet paprika

4 (poached) eggs

1 pinch sugar

1 teaspoon white vinegar

Water

2 (chopped) Roma tomatoes

1 (chopped finely) red onion, small

1 cup fresh chopped cilantro, remove stems

1/2 cup feta, crumbled

Preparation

1. Add 1 1/2 tablespoon olive oil into a big cast iron skillet over med-high heat.

2. Add the potatoes, garlic and chopped onions into the oil.

3. Sprinkle with pepper and salt and stir cook until potatoes are softened, for 5-7 minutes.

4. Add asparagus, chickpeas, spices, a pinch of pepper and salt and mix until combined.

5. Cook for 5-7 more minutes before adjusting heat to low heat.

6. Stir frequently while the hash is kept warm.

7. In the meantime, add water into an average pot and bring to a steady simmering.

8. Add 1 teaspoon vinegar into the simmering water.

9. Crack eggs into a bowl. Lightly stir the vinegar water mixture while you slowly slip the eggs in.

10. Cook eggs in vinegar water for 3 minutes before removing to a kitchen towel until lightly drained.

11. Sprinkle pepper and salt over cooked eggs.

12. Serve warmed potato hash with parsley, feta, tomatoes and onion.

13. Top each plate with the eggs.

Nutritional Information/Serving

Calories 535 kcal, Protein 26.6g, Total Carbs 34.5g, Sodium 295.8mg, Total Fat 20.8g

Mediterranean Breakfast Donuts

Preparation Time: 20 minutes

Cook Time: 15 minutes

Serves: 24 servings

Ingredients

1 teaspoon sugar

1 teaspoon instant yeast

2 cups flour, all-purpose

1 1/4 cup (divided) lukewarm water

Canola oil

1 tablespoon corn starch

Syrup

1 cup honey

1 cup sugar

1 stick cinnamon

1 3/4 cup water

1/4 teaspoon lime juice

Preparation

1. Add sugar and yeast into 1/4 cup lukewarm water, stir to combine and let sit until yeast mixture foams.

2. Add corn starch, flour, 1 cup lukewarm water and the yeast mixture and stir until wholly combined.

3. Place a damp cloth over bowl until covered and let sit for 2 hours in a warm area until it rises.

Note: Use a wooden spoon to remove air bubbles from dough by stirring three to four times during the resting time.

4. Once ready, add canola oil into a small heavy saucepan over med-high heat, about 1/3 of the way.

5. Work in batches, scoop dough into the heated oil with 2 oiled spoons.

6. Once cooked, dough will float to the surface with the base side a golden-brown color.

7. Turn dough, cook and remove swiftly to a big parchment paper lined tray until drained.

8. Repeat process until no dough remains.

9. Add cinnamon stick, water, honey and sugar into a small pot over high heat and bring to boiling while you stir until sugar is dissolved.

10. Adjust to low heat and cook until syrup is thickened, for some minutes.

11. Take pot off heat, add the lime juice and stir until incorporated.

12. Work in batches, drop donuts into the hot honey syrup until wholly coated.

13. Move syrup coated donuts to plate and dribble with any extra syrup.

14. Serve and enjoy.

Nutritional Information/Serving

Calories 200 kcal, Protein 1.2g, Total Carbs 29.5g, Sodium 2.2mg, Total Fat 9.2g

Greek Yogurt Parfait

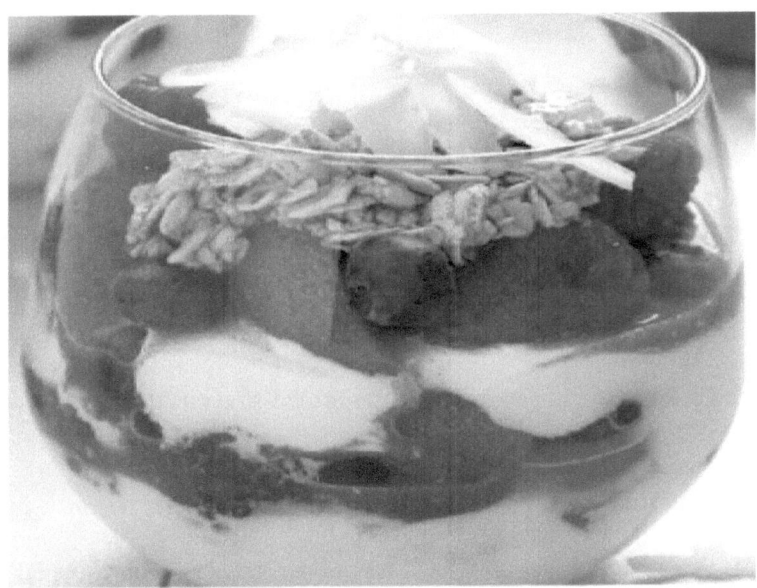

Preparation Time: 5 minutes

Cook Time: 0 minutes

Serves: 6 servings

Ingredients

1 1/4 cup Greek yogurt, low-fat

2 cups homemade or store-bought pumpkin puree

1 teaspoon vanilla extract

3–4 tablespoons whipped low-fat ricotta cheese

2 1/2 tablespoon brown sugar

2 tablespoons molasses

1 pinch nutmeg

1 1/2–2 teaspoon cinnamon

Garnish with

walnuts, chopped

Chocolate chips

Preparation

1. Add Greek yogurt, pumpkin puree and every other ingredient into a big bowl, excluding the garnishes.

2. Whisk until well combined and a smooth texture forms, using a whisk.

3. Check taste, adjust cinnamon or brown sugar as desired and whisk until fully combined.

4. Pour into small jars, seal the lid and refrigerate for a short while.

5. Dribble molasses over each jar or bowl and top with chopped walnuts and chocolate chips.

Nutritional Information/Serving

Calories 102 kcal, Protein 0.8g, Total Carbs 15.6g, Sodium 24.5mg, Total Fat 1.5g

Mediterranean Apple Galette

Preparation Time: 15 minutes

Cook Time: 60 minutes

Serves: 6 servings

Ingredients (dough)

1/2 cup corn flour

2 cups flour, all-purpose

1/2 teaspoon salt

1 teaspoon sugar

1/2 cup ice water

12 tablespoons (cubed) unsalted butter

Topping

1/2 cup apple cider vinegar

2 (peeled, cored and sliced into 1/4" slices) fuji apples, large

1/2 teaspoon cinnamon, ground

2 tablespoons brown sugar

Egg wash = 1 tablespoon water + 1 egg, beaten together

1/2 teaspoon nutmeg, ground

2 tablespoons (cubed) unsalted butter

Preparation

1. Add salt, sugar, corn flour and all-purpose flour into a bowl and whisk until combined.

2. Add half of the butter into the flour mixture and work dough until a rough meal consistency is reached, using clean hands.

3. Add the other half of the butter and work into the dough.

4. Add ice water and keep working until dough is consistent.

5. Press dough until flattened and round, and wrap until wholly covered with plastic.

6. Place wrapped dough into a refrigerator and let sit for 30 minutes.

7. Heat up oven to 400°F.

8. Add slices of apples into a deep bowl and top with apple cider vinegar and let sit for 15 minutes.

9. Add nutmeg, cinnamon and sugar into the apple slices and combine.

10. Lightly flour a flat work surface, add chilled dough and roll out until dough forms a big rectangle, using a rolling pin.

11. Prepare a big parchment paper lined baking sheet and add the dough cautiously.

12. Get rid of the apple cider vinegar and transfer apples into the baking sheet on top over dough.

Tip: Lay apple slices in 2 overlying lines and leave 1" room around the dough.

13. Fold the dough edges over topping until a border is created.

14. Coat dough border with the egg wash and blotch the topping with cubed butter.

15. Transfer baking sheet into the preheated oven and bake for 30 minutes.

16. Spin the baking sheet until position is changed and bake until the apple pie crust becomes golden brown, for 30 more minutes.

17. Remove baking sheet from the oven and let galette sit until cooled before you slice.

18. Serve with favorite syrup and enjoy.

Nutritional Information/Serving

Calories 642 kcal, Protein 7.7g, Total Carbs 79.9g, Sodium 220.4mg, Total Fat 32.2g

Creamy Peaches Baguette

Preparation Time: 10 minutes

Cook Time: 20 minutes

Serves: 10 servings

Ingredients

6 ounces softened cream cheese

1/3 cup Greek yogurt

1/3 cup sugar

1 generous tablespoon orange zest

1 pinch cinnamon, ground

1 pinch nutmeg, ground

3 tablespoons orange juice

3 (cored and sliced thinly into wedges) peaches

1/4 cup pecan halves, coarsely chopped

10 (toasted) crostini (French baguette slices)

Serve with

Honey

Preparation

1. Add cinnamon, nutmeg, sugar, zest of orange, cream cheese and Greek yogurt into the food processor and process until a fluffy and smooth consistency is reached.

2. Pour the whipped yogurt mixture into a bowl, place lid over bowl and transfer into a refrigerator for an hour.

3. Heat up oven to 425°F.

4. Pour orange juice and add the peaches into a bowl and toss until coated.

5. Casually pat dry the peaches and transfer onto a parchment paper lined baking sheet.

6. Transfer baking sheet into the preheated oven and bake for 20-25 minutes.

7. Spread the whipped yogurt mixture over toasted baguette slices.

8. Add roasted peach slices and chopped pecans over the yogurt spread on each baguette slice.

9. Dribble with honey and serve.

Nutritional Information/Serving

Calories 200 kcal, Protein 4.2g, Total Carbs 28.4g, Sodium 57.3mg, Total Fat 8.5g

Cheesy Cilantro Casserole

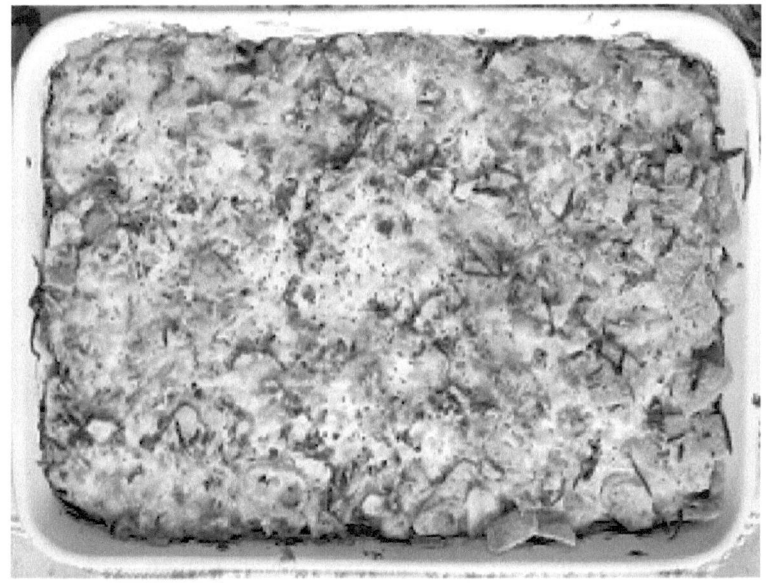

Preparation Time: 15 minutes

Cook Time: 35 minutes

Serves: 6 servings

Ingredients

1 (chopped) tomato, large

10 ounces (coarsely chopped and cook in a microwave according to directions on the package) artichokes, frozen

1 cup (remove stems and chop leaves coarsely) fresh cilantro

1 (chopped) shallot, large

1 1/4 cup feta cheese, crumbled

1 cup (remove stems and chop leaves coarsely) fresh mint leaves

6 slices (cut into 1/2" pieces) fresh toast

1/2 cup Parmesan cheese, ground

6 eggs

1 1/2 cup milk

1/4 teaspoon nutmeg, ground

1/2 teaspoon baking powder

Salt and pepper, as necessary

1 teaspoon hot paprika

Preparation

1. Heat up oven to 375°F.

2. Transfer the toast pieces into a big bowl and let sit until needed.

3. Add pepper, salt, hot paprika, nutmeg, baking powder, eggs and milk into a second bowl and whisk until combined.

4. Pour egg milk into the bowl with toast.

5. Add the cheese, herbs and veggies into the egg mixture and stir until combined.

6. Pour mixture into an oven secure baking dish and transfer into the preheated oven.

7. Bake until well-cooked for 35 minutes.

8. Serve and enjoy.

Nutritional Information/Serving

Calories 353 kcal, Protein 22g, Total Carbs 35g, Sodium 542.6mg, Total Fat 16g

Barley Raspberry Compote

Preparation Time: 10 minutes

Cook Time: 45 minutes

Serves: 6 servings

Ingredients

3 cups water

1 1/2 cups (rinsed with cold water and well drained) pearl barley

3 tablespoons (divided) sugar

1 1/2 cup milk

1/3 cup coconut chips

1/4 teaspoon salt

1/3 cup pistachios, shelled

1/3 cup almonds, sliced

Compote

6 oz fresh raspberries

6 ounces fresh strawberries

3/4 cup water

3/4 cup sugar

1 teaspoon vanilla extract

1 tablespoon lime juice

1/4 scant tsp cardamom, ground

Preparation

1. Add milk, salt, 2 tablespoons sugar, water and barley into an average heavy saucepan over high heat, combine and bring to boiling.

2. Adjust to low heat, place lid over saucepan and cook until cooking juice is absorbed and the barley is softened, for 45 minutes.

3. Add the reserved 1 tablespoon sugar, pistachios, almonds and coconut chips into a small bowl, combine and let sit until needed.

4. Add cardamom, vanilla extract, lime juice, water, sugar and the berries into a heavy saucepan over high heat and bring to boiling.

5. Adjust heat to med-low heat, stir and simmer for 12-15 minutes.

6. Take saucepan off heat and let sit until cooled.

7. Serve barley with the compote, garnished with the almond mixture.

8. Serve and enjoy.

Nutritional Information/Serving

Calories 505 kcal, Protein 10g, Total Carbs 90.2g, Sodium 134.7mg, Total Fat 13.5g

LUNCH

Kofta Lettuce Wraps

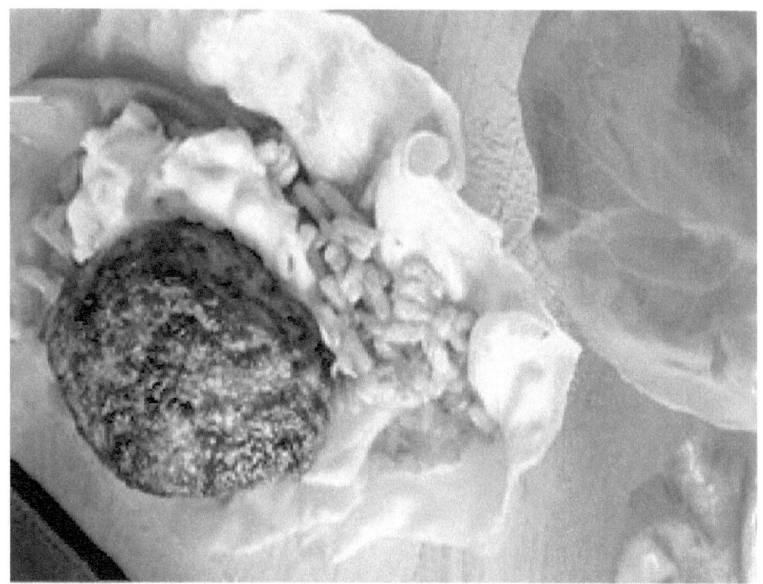

Preparation Time: 10 minutes

Cook Time: 23 minutes

Serves: 4 servings

Ingredients

8 oz. ground beef

1 (1 oz.) {torn} slice bread, whole-grain

5 tbsps (divided) red onion, grated

6 oz. lean ground lamb

1 tbsp fresh chopped rosemary

2 tbsps fresh chopped cilantro

1/2 tsp allspice, ground

1/2 tsp cinnamon, ground

3/4 tsp (divided) salt

1 egg, large

1 tbsp (divided) olive oil

1/2 tsp (divided) black pepper, freshly ground

3 tbsps English cucumber, diced

3/4 cup Greek yogurt, 2% low-fat

1 tsp paprika

1 (8.8 oz.) brown rice, precooked

12 lettuce leaves

Preparation

1. Add torn bread into a food processor and pulse until a big crumb consistency is reached.

2. Add egg, allspice, cinnamon, rosemary, cilantro, onion, lamb, beef and bread into a big bowl and combine.

3. Sprinkle 1/4 tsp pepper and 1/2 tsp salt over beef mixture and lightly mix until combined.

4. Form beef mixture into 12 (1" thick) patties.

5. Add 1 tsp olive oil into a big nonstick skillet over med-high heat.

6. Swirl skillet until pan is coated and add the patties.

7. Cook patties until well-cooked for 2 1/2 minutes per side.

8. Add the remaining 3 tbsps onion, cucumber, the remaining 1 tsp pepper, the remaining 1/4 tsp salt and the yogurt into a big bowl and stir until well combined.

9. Cook the rice according to instructions on the package, stir in paprika and 2 tsps olive oil and toss lightly until well combined.

10. Split yogurt, patties and rice into lettuce leaves, wrap and serve.

Nutritional Information/Serving

Calories 408 kcal, Carbs 27g, Fat 26g, Protein 26g, Sodium 592mg

Zucchini Turkey Kofta

Preparation Time: 10 minutes

Cook Time: 13 minutes

Serves: 4 servings

Ingredients

1/4 cup breadcrumbs, dry

1/2 cup (divided) tzatziki, store-bought

5 tbsps (divided) fresh chopped rosemary

1/4 cup onion, grated

5/8 tsp (divided) salt

1 tsp ground cumin

1/8 tsp red pepper, ground

3/8 tsp (divided) black pepper

4 tsps (divided) olive oil

1 lb. turkey, ground

Cooking spray

4 (halved lengthways) zucchini

Preparation

1. Heat up broiler to high heat.

2. Add red pepper, 1/4 tsp black pepper, 1/2 tsp salt, cumin, 3 tbsps rosemary, onion, breadcrumbs and 1/4 cup tzatziki into a bowl and whisk until combined.

3. Add ground turkey into the mixture and mix until combined with clean hands before forming mixture into 8 patties.

4. Add 2 tsps olive oil into a nonstick skillet over med-heat.

5. Add patties into the heated skillet and cook until well cooked, for 4 minutes per side.

6. In the meantime, coat a baking pan with cooking spray and add the zucchini with the open side up.

7. Brush zucchini insides with the remaining 2 tsps olive oil and season with 1/8 tsp black pepper and 1/8 tsp salt.

8. Broil seasoned zucchini until softened, for about 5 minutes.

9. Split zucchini and turkey kofta into serving platters, topped with the remaining rosemary.

10. Serve with the reserved tzatziki.

Nutritional Information/Serving

Calories 418 kcal, Carbs 22g, Fat 22g, Protein 34g, Sodium 541mg

Lime Oregano Shrimp Pasta

Preparation Time: 10 minutes

Cook Time: 11 minutes

Serves: 4 servings

Ingredients

8 oz. spaghetti, uncooked

3 qts. water

1/4 cup fresh chopped oregano

1 lb. shrimp, large (peeled & deveined)

2 tbsps olive oil

3 tbsps capers, drained

1/2 tsp salt

2 tbsps lime juice

2 cups baby spinach

Preparation

1. Add 3 qts water into a Dutch oven and bring to boiling.

2. Add pasta into the boiling water and cook for 8 minutes until just cooked.

3. Add the prepared shrimp into the pot and cook until pasta is al dente and the shrimp is well cooked, for about 3 more minutes.

4. Drain water from pasta and transfer shrimp/pasta mixture into a big bowl.

5. Add salt, lime juice, olive oil, capers and oregano into the pasta mixture and stir until combined.

6. Split spinach among 4 serving plates and top evenly with the shrimp pasta mixture.

7. Serve and enjoy.

Nutritional Information/Serving

Calories 359 kcal, Carbs 47g, Fat 9g, Protein 22g, Sodium 1347mg

Greek Chicken Burgers

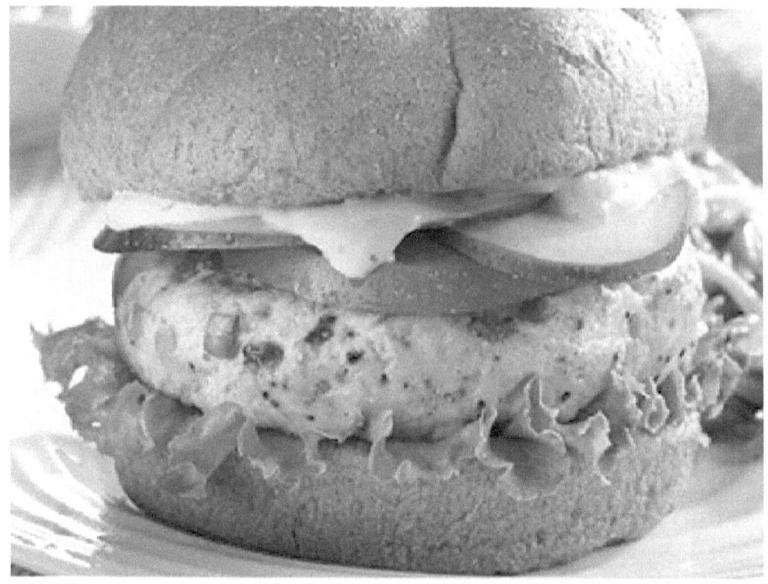

Preparation Time: 5 minutes

Cook Time: 16 minutes

Serves: 4 servings

Ingredients

1 cup red onion, chopped

1 egg white, large

1/2 cup breadcrumbs, dry

3/4 cup fresh chopped parsley

2 tbsps lime juice

1/3 cup feta cheese, crumbled

1 lb. chicken, ground

1 tsp dill, dried

4 (1.5 oz.) (split in halves) hamburger buns

Cooking spray

1 (7 oz.) bottle (drain and cut into 1" strips) roasted red bell peppers

Preparation

1. Add egg white into a big bowl and whisk until lightly beaten.

2. Add onion, bread crumbs, parsley, lime juice, ground chicken, feta cheese, and dill into the egg white mixture and stir until wholly combined.

3. Shape ground chicken mixture into 4 even (1/2" thick) patties.

4. Coat a big nonstick skillet with cooking spray and place over med-high heat.

5. Add patties into the heated skillet and cook until well-cooked for 8 minutes per side.

6. Add the cooked burger patties on each hamburger bottom half.

7. Split roasted red pepper slices among each burger and top with each hamburger top half.

8. Serve and enjoy.

Nutritional Information/Serving

Calories 426 kcal, Sodium 790mg, Carbs 40g, Protein 30.5g, Fat 15.7g

Bulgur Turkey Salad

Preparation Time: 10 minutes

Cook Time: 20 minutes

Serves: 4 servings

Ingredients

2/3 cup bulgur

1 1/3 cups water

1 lb. turkey breast cutlets

Cooking spray

1/2 tsp black pepper

1 tsp (divided) salt

2 cups cherry tomatoes, halved

4 cups arugula, packed

3 tbsps olive oil

2 cups peaches, sliced

2 tbsps rice vinegar

Preparation

1. Add bulgur and 1 1/3 cups water into a small saucepan over high heat and bring to boiling.

2. Adjust heat to med-low, place lid over saucepan and simmer the bulgur mixture for 10 minutes.

3. Drain water and rinse bulgur under cold running water.

4. Transfer well drained bulgur onto paper towels.

5. In the meantime, spray cooking spray over a grill pan and heat up to high heat.

6. Season turkey with pepper and 1/2 tsp salt and transfer into the prepared grill pan.

7. Grill turkey until well-cooked for 6-7 minutes.

Note: turn turkey every now and then for even cooking.

8. Let turkey sit on a cutting board until cooled and slice into strips against the grain.

9. Add the peaches, tomatoes, arugula and bulgur into a big bowl.

10. Add vinegar, olive oil and the reserved 1/2 tsp salt into the bulgur bowl and toss until combined.

11. Split mixture into serving plates and top with turkey.

12. Serve and enjoy.

Nutritional Information/Serving

Calories 364 kcal, Sodium 547mg, Carbs 30g, Protein 31g, Fat 14g

Cheese Spring Salad

Preparation Time: 10 minutes

Cook Time: 6 minutes

Serves: 4 servings

Ingredients

1 1/2 cups (cut into 1" pieces) fresh asparagus

8 cups water

3/4 tsp (divided) salt

1 cup green peas, frozen

1 tbsp rosemary, finely chopped

1 tbsp cilantro, finely chopped

1 tsp lemon zest

1 (3 ounces) goat cheese log

1 tsp mustard, whole-grain

2 tbsps lemon juice

1 tsp basil, finely chopped

1 tsp honey

2 1/2 tbsps olive oil

1/4 tsp black pepper

1 cup radishes, sliced thin

6 oz. fresh baby spinach

1 tbsp rosemary

1/4 cup unsalted almonds, roasted

Preparation

1. Add 8 cups water into an average stockpot over high heat and bring to boiling.

2. Add the peas and asparagus into the boiling water and cook for 2-3 minutes until softened.

3. Drain water and immediately dip the peas and asparagus into an ice bath to stop the cooking process.

4. Drain water from the asparagus mixture and move into a paper towel line baking sheet.

5. Season pea and asparagus with 1/4 tsp salt.

6. Place a 12-by-12" plastic wrap on a flat work surface and scatter rosemary and cilantro in the center of the plastic wrap.

7. Roll the cheese log in the rosemary mixture until coated and keep rolling until the plastic square is wrapped around the cheese.

8. Carefully roll until log is 4" long before slicing into eight (1/2" thick) rounds.

Note: Get rid of the plastic wraps after slicing.

9. Add 1/2 tsp salt, pepper, chopped basil, honey, mustard, lemon juice and lemon zest into a bowl and whisk until combined.

10. Gradually add while whisking until fully incorporated.

11. Add spinach into the lemon dressing mixture and toss until combined and coated.

12. Add the radishes, peas and asparagus into the spinach mixture and combine.

13. Serve topped with rosemary, cheese and almonds.

Nutritional Information/Serving

Calories 245 kcal, Sodium 541mg, Carbs 14g, Protein 10g, Fat 18g

Feta Turkey Spinach Salad

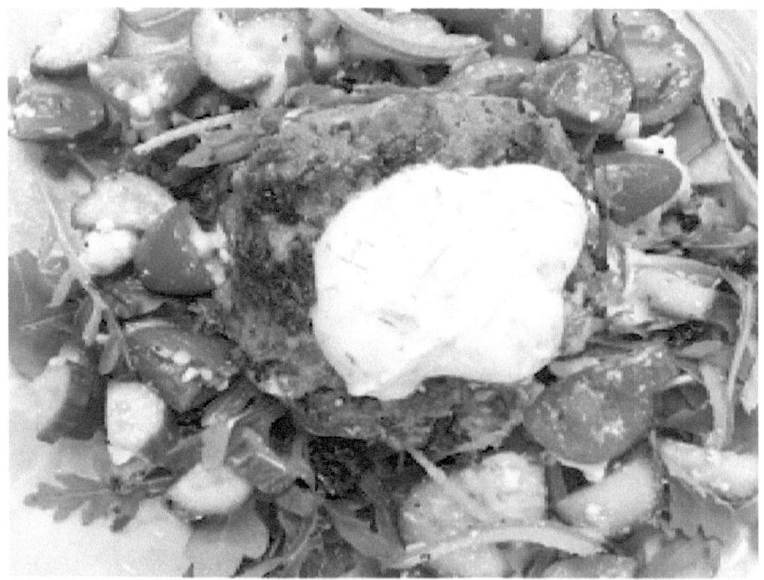

Preparation Time: 10 minutes

Cook Time: 8 minutes

Serves: 4 servings

Ingredients

1/2 tsp lime rind, grated

1/4 cup chicken broth, reduced-sodium, no-fat

1 tbsp balsamic vinegar

1 tbsp lime juice

1 tsp garlic, minced

1 tsp sugar

1 tsp olive oil

1 tsp Dijon mustard

Cooking spray

1/2 tsp salt

1/4 tsp black pepper

1 lb. turkey breast, skinless, boneless

1 1/4 cups (slice into 1" pieces) yellow bell pepper

1 1/2 cups red onion, chopped

1 (15.5 oz.) can {drained} chickpeas

1/2 cup feta cheese, crumbled

1 (7-ounce) package baby spinach, prewashed

Preparation

1. Add salt, olive oil, mustard, garlic, sugar, balsamic vinegar, lime juice, lime rind and broth into a bowl and whisk until combined.

2. Coat a big nonstick skillet with cooking spray and place over med-high heat.

3. Sprinkle black pepper over turkey until evenly coated.

4. Add seasoned turkey into the heated skillet and cook for 4 minutes.

5. Add onions into the turkey mixture, flip turkey and stir cook until onion is softened and turkey is well cooked for 4 more minutes.

6. Remove turkey into a plate, let sit until cooled and slice into 1/2" thick slices.

7. Add spinach, chickpeas, cheese, bell pepper, onion and turkey into a big bowl and toss until wholly combined.

8. Dribble lime dressing over salad and toss again until coated.

9. Serve and enjoy.

Nutritional Information/Serving

Calories 371 kcal, Carbs 34g, Fat 9g, Protein 46g, Sodium 971mg

Turkish Beef Meatballs with Pita

Preparation Time: 12 minutes

Cook Time: 8 minutes

Serves: 4 servings

Ingredients

1/3 cup breadcrumbs, dry

1/2 cup white onion, chopped

2 tbsps tomato paste

1/4 cup fresh chopped rosemary

1/2 tsp salt

1 tsp garlic, minced

1/4 tsp cinnamon, ground

1/2 tsp cumin, ground

1/8 tsp allspice, ground

1/4 tsp red pepper, ground

1 (beaten lightly) egg white, large

1 lb. lean ground beef

8 (1/4" thick) plum tomato slices

Cooking spray

1/4 cup plain yogurt

4 (6") pitas, halved

Preparation

1. Heat up broiler.

2. Add the egg white, ground beef, allspice, red pepper, ground cinnamon, cumin, salt, minced garlic, tomato paste, fresh chopped rosemary, bread crumbs and white onion into a big bowl and stir to combine.

3. Split and shape mixture into 8(2") patties.

4. Prepare a cooking spray coated baking pan.

5. Add patties into the prepared pan and broil until cooked as desired, for 4 minutes per side.

6. Top each pita half with 1 patty and 1 tomato slice and top with 1 1/2 tsps plain yogurt until evenly coated.

Nutritional Information/Serving

Calories 480 kcal, Carbs 50g, Fat 14g, Protein 35g, Sodium 791mg

Tomato Tuna Steaks

Preparation Time: 12 minutes

Cook Time: 8 minutes

Serves: 4 servings

Ingredients

1/2 tsp (divided) salt

4 (6 oz.) ahi tuna steaks

1/8 tsp black pepper

1/2 tsp coriander, ground

1 1/2 cups tomato, chopped and seeded

Cooking spray

3 tbsps fresh chopped cilantro

1/4 cup green onions, chopped

1 tbsp olive oil

1 tbsp (drained) capers

1/2 tsp garlic, minced

1 tbsp lime juice

12 pitted kalamata olives, chopped

Preparation

1. Coat a big nonstick skillet with cooking spray and place over med-high heat.

2. Season tuna steaks with pepper, coriander and 1/4 tsp salt until wholly covered.

3. Add the seasoned tuna steaks into the pan and cook until well-cooked for 4 minutes per side.

4. In the meantime, add the tomato, the reserved 1/4 tsp salt and every other ingredient into a bowl and combine.

5. Serve fish with tomato sauce.

Nutritional Information/Serving

Calories 301 kcal, Carbs 16g, Fat 9g, Protein 47g, Sodium 640mg

Mediterranean Kofta Kebab

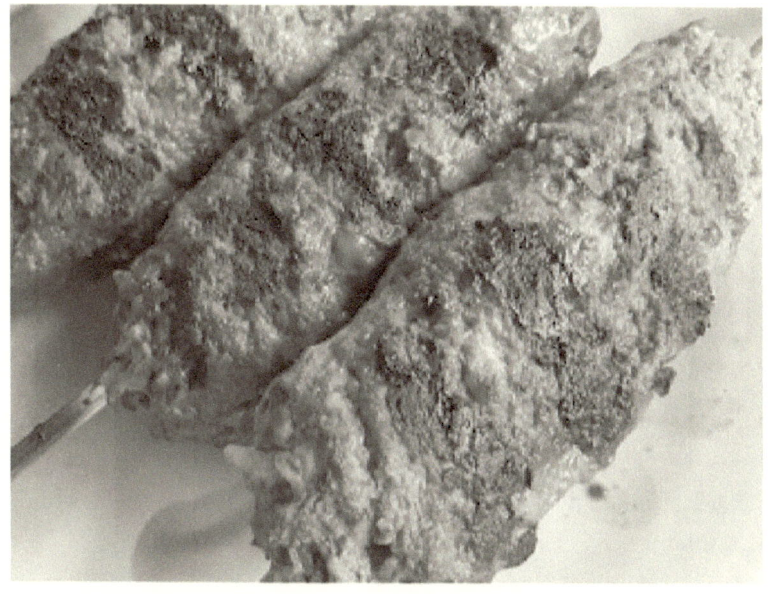

Preparation Time: 20 minutes

Cook Time: 8 minutes

Serves: 10 servings

Ingredients

2 garlic cloves

1 (quartered) yellow onion, medium

1 pound beef, ground

1 (remove stems) whole bunch cilantro

1 (toasted and soaked until wholly softened in water) bread slice

1/2 pound lamb, ground

1 1/2 teaspoon allspice, ground

Salt and pepper

1/2 teaspoon green cardamom, ground

1/2 teaspoon cayenne pepper

1/2 teaspoon nutmeg, ground

1/2 teaspoon lemon pepper seasoning

1/2 teaspoon paprika

Preparation

1. Place 10 bamboo skewers into a bowl with water for an hour and soak.

2. Remove skewers just before prepping your meal.

3. Grease the grates of a gas grill lightly and heat up to med-high heat for 20 minutes.

4. Add cilantro, garlic and onion into a food processor and process until chopped.

5. Squeeze out water from the bread until no water remains.

6. Add spices, bread, lamb and beef into the food processor mixture and process until a paste-like consistency is reached.

7. Transfer mixture into a big bowl and form into 1" sized balls.

8. Thread meatballs on the soaked bamboo skewers until no meat remains.

9. Prepare a parchment paper lined baking tray and add the kofta kebabs.

10. Transfer kebabs onto the prepared grill and grill for 4 minutes on a side.

11. Flip kebabs and grill for 3-4 more minutes.

12. Serve as desired and enjoy.

Nutritional Information/Serving

Calories 247 kcal, Protein 19.2g, Total Carbs 27g, Sodium 236.9mg, Total Fat 7.8g

Stuffed Peppers

Preparation Time: 15 minutes

Cook Time: 50 minutes

Serves: 6 servings

Ingredients

1 (chopped) yellow onion, small

Olive oil

Salt and pepper

1/2 pound beef, ground

1/2 teaspoon garlic powder

1/2 teaspoon allspice

1/2 cup cilantro, chopped

1 cup chickpeas, canned or cooked

1/2 teaspoon sweet paprika

1 cup (soaked for 15 minutes in water and drained) short grain rice

2 1/4 cup water

3 tablespoons tomato sauce

3/4 cup chicken broth

6 (remove tops and core) bell peppers

Preparation

1. Add 1 tablespoon olive oil into an average heavy pot.

2. Add chopped onions into the oil and cook until golden.

3. Add ground beef into the mixture and stir cook until wholly browned on med-high heat.

4. Sprinkle garlic powder, all spice, pepper and salt over beef mixture.

5. Add chickpeas into the beef mixture, stir to combine and cook for few minutes until warmed.

6. Add tomato sauce, paprika, rice and cilantro into the mixture and stir until combined.

7. Add water into the mixture and bring to a rolling simmer.

Note: Cooking juices will be reduced by 1/2.

8. Adjust heat to low heat, place lid over pot and cook until rice is just soft and well cooked, for 15-20 minutes.

9. In the meantime, prepare a gas grill set to med-high.

10. Add bell peppers to prepared grill, cover peppers and grill for 10-15 minutes.

11. Flip peppers every now and then to ensure even cooking.

12. Once peppers are wholly grilled, take off the grill and let sit to cool.

13. Heat up oven to 350°F.

14. Prepare a 3/4 cup broth filled baking dish.

15. Layer the grilled bell peppers with the close-side down into the prepared baking dish.

16. Scoop the rice mixture into the peppers until wholly filled.

17. Place aluminum foil over baking dish until tightly covered and transfer into the preheated oven.

18. Bake peppers for 20-30 minutes until desired doneness is reached.

19. Serve garnished with cilantro.

Nutritional Information/Serving

Calories 281 kcal, Protein 14.5g, Total Carbs 44.4g, Sodium 37.7mg, Total Fat 4.8g

Colorful Baked Veggie with Eggs

Preparation Time: 10 minutes

Cook Time: 20 minutes

Serves: 6 servings

Ingredients

1 (remove core and slice thinly) orange bell pepper

1 (remove core and slice thinly) green bell pepper

1 (halve and slice thinly) medium red onion

1 (remove core and slice thinly) red bell pepper

1 teaspoon (divided) harissa

Salt and black pepper

1 teaspoon chili pepper

1 teaspoon cumin, ground

6 big eggs

Olive oil

1 diced Roma tomato

Fresh chopped cilantro

Preparation

1. Heat up oven to 400°F.

2. Add chili pepper, cumin, harissa, pepper, salt, red onions and all the sliced peppers into a big bowl.

3. Dribble olive oil over veggies and toss until combined.

4. Spread onion/pepper mixture in a single layer into a big baking sheet.

5. Transfer baking sheet into the preheated oven and bake for 15 minutes.

6. Take out baking sheet from the oven, make six cavities on the baked veggies.

7. Crack an egg into each veggie cavity and make sure the yoke remains whole.

8. Place baking sheet into the oven and bake until eggs are set for about 8 minutes.

9. Take out baking sheet from the oven and season eggs as desired.

10. Sprinkle feta, diced tomatoes, chopped cilantro and harissa over egg and veggies.

11. Serve at once and enjoy.

Nutritional Information/Serving

Calories 111 kcal, Protein 6.9g, Total Carbs 4.5g, Sodium 267.4mg, Total Fat 7.3g

Lettuce Wraps with Lamb

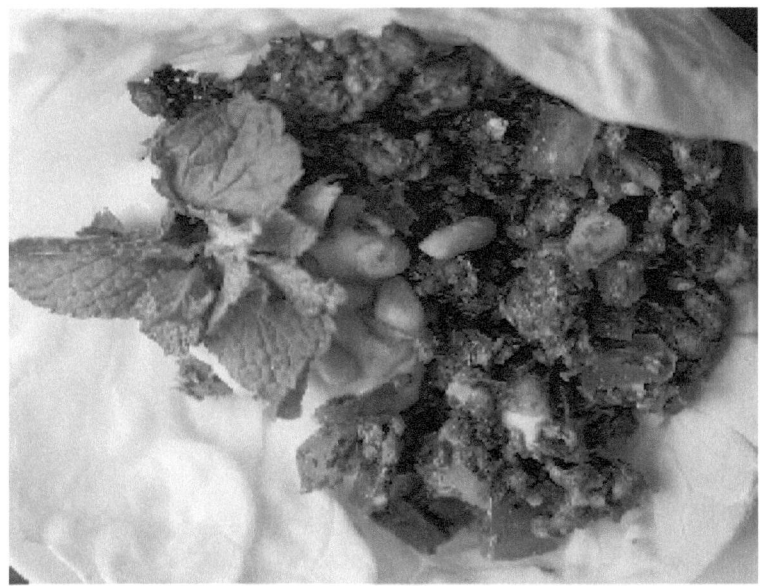

Preparation Time: 15 minutes

Cook Time: 5 minutes

Serves: 4 servings

Ingredients

1 cup onion, chopped finely

2 tsps olive oil

1 tsp cinnamon, ground

2 tsps fresh garlic, minced

1/4 tsp black pepper, freshly ground

3/4 tsp salt

1/2 cup fresh cilantro, chopped

6 oz. ground lamb, lean

1/2 cup cucumber, chopped

1/2 cup tomato, chopped

1/4 cup red pepper hummus

1/4 cup Greek yogurt, plain fat-free

2 tbsps chopped basil

8 lettuce leaves

1 tbsp toasted pine nuts

Preparation

1. Add olive oil into a big skillet over high heat.

2. Swirl skillet until wholly coated.

3. Add the lamb, pepper, salt, cinnamon, garlic and onion into the heated pan and saute until ground lamb is well cooked, for 5 minutes.

4. Add cucumber, tomato and cilantro into an average bowl and stir until combined.

5. Add the ground lamb mixture into the cucumber bowl and mix until evenly distributed.

6. Add humus and yogurt into a separate bowl and combine.

7. Fill each lettuce lead with 1/4 cup of the ground lamb mixture.

8. Add 1 tbsp of the yogurt mixture over lamb mixture and evenly sprinkle with pine nuts and chopped basil.

9. Serve and enjoy.

Nutritional Information/Serving

Calories 224 kcal, Carbs 14g, Fat 11g, Protein 18g, Sodium 543mg

Yummy Greek Scampi

Preparation Time: 10 minutes

Cook Time: 23 minutes

Serves: 4 servings

Ingredients

4 minced garlic cloves

1 tbsp olive oil

1/8 tsp salt

1/4 cup (divided) fresh chopped cilantro

1 1/4 lb. (peeled & deveined) shrimp, large

4 (14.5 oz.) cans {drained & chopped} whole peeled tomatoes, no-salt-added

1 1/2 tbsps fresh lime juice

3/4 cup feta cheese, crumbled

1/4 tsp black pepper, freshly ground

Preparation

1. Heat up oven to 400°F.

2. Add olive oil into a big Dutch oven over med-heat.

3. Swirl pot with oil until coated.

4. Add garlic into the heated pot and stir cook for 30 seconds.

5. Add tomatoes, salt and 2 tbsps cilantro into the pot, adjust heat to low and simmer mixture for 7 minutes.

6. Add shrimp into the pot and cook for 5 more minutes.

7. Empty shrimp mixture into a 7-by-11" glass baking dish and top with feta evenly.

8. Transfer baking sheet into the preheated oven and bake for 10 minutes.

9. Serve, topped with pepper, lime juice, cilantro and the reserved 2 tbsps cilantro.

Nutritional Information/Serving

Calories 301 kcal, Sodium 569mg, Carbs 13.1g, Protein 34.4g, Fat 10.4g

Middle Eastern Chicken Burgers

Preparation Time: 10 minutes

Cook Time: 10 minutes

Serves: 4 servings

Ingredients

1/4 cup mayo

1 lb. ground chicken, 93% lean

1 tsp cumin, ground

2 tsps basil, dried

1/4 tsp (divided) black pepper

1/4 tsp salt

1/3 cup whole-milk Greek yogurt, plain

Cooking spray

1 tbsp lime juice

1/3 cup kalamata olives, chopped

2 cups arugula

4 hamburger buns, whole wheat

1/2 cup red onion, sliced thin

1/2 cup cucumber, sliced

Preparation

1. Add 1/8 tsp pepper, salt, cumin, basil, mayo and ground chicken into a bowl, combine and form into 4 even patties.

2. Casually coat a big cast iron skillet with cooking spray and place over high heat.

3. Add the chicken patties into the heated skillet and cook for 4-5 minutes on each side until an inserted thermometer reads 165°F.

4. Add the reserved 1/8 tsp pepper, lime juice, olives and yogurt into a bowl and combine.

5. Coat the insides of the upper and bottom hamburger buns with yogurt mixture.

6. Top each bottom halves of the buns with the red onion, cucumber, cooked patties and arugula and top filling with each upper bun.

7. Serve and enjoy.

Nutritional Information/Serving

Calories 375 kcal, Sodium 699mg, Carbs 28g, Protein 29g, Fat 17g

Greek Olive Turkey Salad

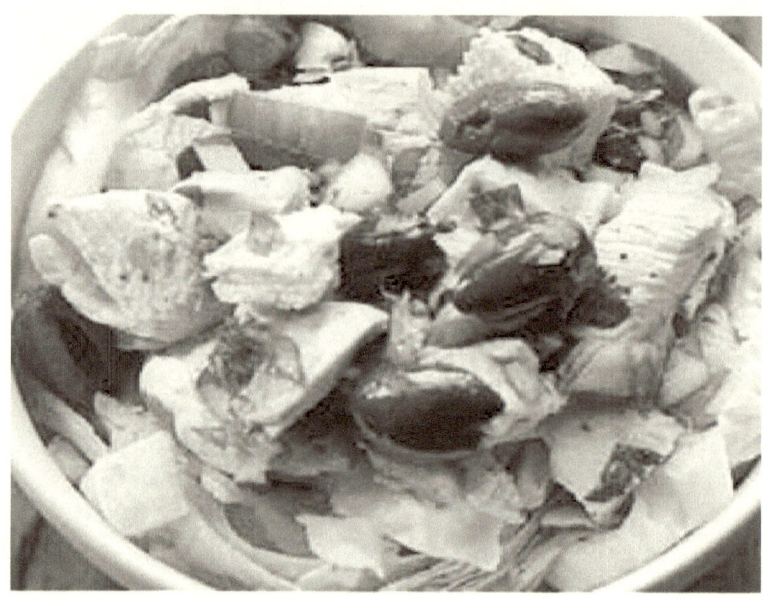

Preparation Time: 10 minutes

Cook Time: 10 minutes

Serves: 4 servings

Ingredients

1/2 tsp garlic powder

1 tsp basil, dried

1/2 tsp (divided) salt

3/4 tsp (divided) black pepper

1 lb. (cut into 1" cubes) turkey breast, boneless and skinless

Cooking spray

1 cup plain yogurt, no-fat

5 tsps (divided) lime juice

1 tsp garlic, minced

2 tsps tahini

1 cup English cucumber, peeled and chopped

8 cups romaine lettuce, chopped

6 kalamata olives, pitted and halved

1 cup (halved) grape tomatoes

1/4 cup feta cheese, crumbled

Preparation

1. Add 1/4 tsp salt, 1/2 tsp pepper, garlic powder and basil into a bowl and combine.

2. Coat a nonstick skillet with cooking spray and place over med-high heat.

3. Add herb/spice mix and turkey into the heated pan and cook until turkey is well cooked on both sides.

4. Dribble with 1 tbsp lime juice, stir to coat and remove turkey from the skillet.

5. Add minced garlic, tahini, yogurt, 1/4 tsp pepper, 1/4 tsp salt and 2 tsp lime juice into a small bowl and stir until combined.

6. Add olives, tomatoes, cucumbers and lettuce into a separate bowl and combine.

7. Serve olive salad mixture into serving platters, evenly topped with cheese and turkey mixture.

8. Serve with the yoghurt mixture and enjoy.

Nutritional Information/Serving

Calories 274 kcal, Carbs 14g, Fat 5g, Protein 41g, Sodium 558mg

Cheese Tomato Pizza

Preparation Time: 15 minutes

Cook Time: 8 minutes

Serves: 6 servings

Ingredients

2 tbsps yellow cornmeal

1 (11 oz.) can French bread dough, chilled

1 1/2 lbs. (sliced thin) plum tomatoes

Cooking spray

1 cup (divided) part-skim mozzarella cheese, shredded

1 minced garlic clove

2 oz. (chopped) pancetta

1/4 tsp black pepper

1/4 cup chopped oregano

Preparation

1. Heat up oven to 450ºF.

2. Sprinkle cornmeal over bread dough and place on a baking dish.

3. Press bread dough into a 12" sphere and crease dough edges until a rim is formed.

4. Use cooking spray to casually spray dough top until coated before transferring into the preheated oven.

5. Bake until well-cooked for 8 minutes before removing from the oven.

6. Add slices of tomato on paper towels and top with extra paper towels.

7. Set tomato slices aside for 5 minutes.

8. Scatter 1/2 cup cheese and minced garlic evenly over dough top.

9. Scatter pepper and tomato slices over dough until evenly covered.

10. Scatter the reserved 1/2 cup cheese over bread dough before placing in the preheated oven.

11. Bake pizza for 5 minutes until just cooked.

12. Add chopped pancetta into a nonstick skillet over med-heat.

13. Cook pancetta until crisp and drain.

14. Scatter pancetta over pizza and bake until the crust becomes golden for 1 extra minute.

15. Scatter chopped oregano over pizza and let sit for 2 minutes.

16. Slice pizza into six wedges.

17. Serve and enjoy.

Nutritional Information/Serving

Calories 280 kcal, Carbs 38g, Fat 9g, Protein 10g, Sodium 479mg

Lamb Gremolada

Preparation Time: 10 minutes

Cook Time: 8 minutes

Serves: 4 servings

Ingredients

1/2 tsp cumin, ground

1/2 tsp salt

1/8 tsp cinnamon, ground

1/4 tsp black pepper

Cooking spray

1/4 tsp coriander, ground

8 (4 oz.) {trimmed} lamb loin chops

3 tbsps fresh chopped cilantro

2 tbsps pistachios, finely chopped

1/8 tsp salt

2 tsps lime rind, grated

1 minced garlic clove

Preparation

1. Coat a big nonstick skillet with cooking spray and place over med-high heat.

2. Season lamb evenly with cinnamon, black pepper, coriander, cumin and salt.

3. Add the seasoned lamb into the heated pan and cook until cooked as desired on both sides, for 4 minutes per side.

4. In the meantime, add every other ingredient and pistachio into a bowl and combine.

5. Scatter pistachio mixture over lamb.

6. Serve and enjoy.

Nutritional Information/Serving

Calories 242 kcal, Carbs 5g, Fat 11g, Protein 33g, Sodium 444mg

Turkey Pita Salad

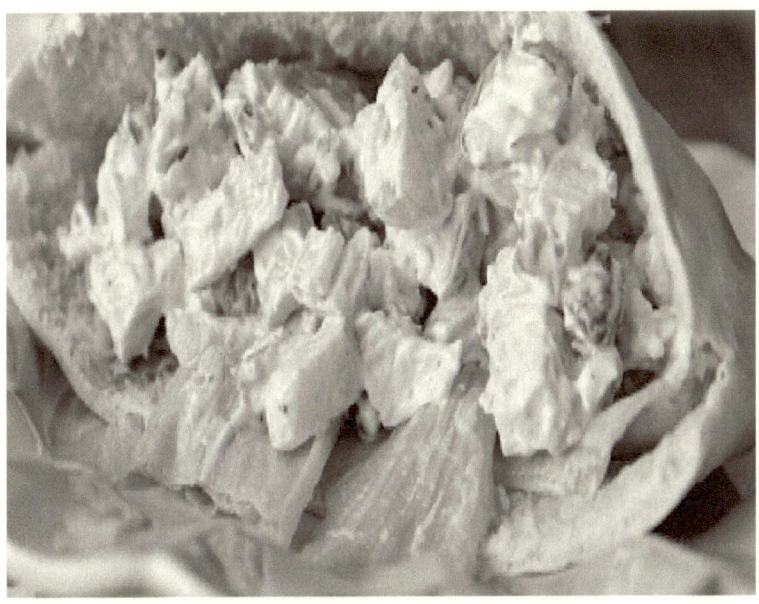

Preparation Time: 8 minutes

Cook Time: 12 minutes

Serves: 4 servings

Ingredients

2 cups fennel bulb, sliced thin

2 (6") pitas

1/2 cup fresh chopped cilantro

1 cup (boneless, skinless) rotisserie turkey breast, shredded

1/2 (half lengthways and slice thin) English cucumber

1/4 cup red onion, sliced

1/4 tsp (divided) black pepper

1/2 tsp (divided) salt

1 tbsp white wine vinegar

1/4 cup lime juice

3 tbsps olive oil

1/2 tsp fresh chopped basil

Preparation

1. Heat up oven to 350°F.

2. Add pitas onto a baking sheet and transfer into the preheated oven.

3. Bake pitas until toasted, for 12 minutes and let sit to cool for a minute.

4. Tear toasted pitas into smaller pieces.

5. Add cucumber, onion, cilantro, turkey, fennel and pita pieces into a bowl and combine.

6. Scatter 1/8 tsp pepper and 1/4 tsp salt over cucumber mixture and stir until combined.

7. Add 1/8 tsp pepper, 1/4 tsp salt, basil, vinegar and lime juice into a bowl and combine.

8. Slowly add olive oil into the lime juice and keep whisking until combined.

9. Dribble lime/olive oil vinaigrette over pita salad and toss until wholly coated.

10. Serve and enjoy.

Nutritional Information/Serving

Calories 373 kcal, Carbs 39g, Fat 19g, Protein 19g, Sodium 846mg

Tomato Pasta Salad

Preparation Time: 10 minutes

Cook Time: 20 minutes

Serves: 4 servings

Ingredients

1 cup French green beans

1 cup penne pasta, uncooked

1 Japanese eggplant, chopped

1 tbsp olive oil

2 pint (halved and divided) cherry tomatoes

1 tbsp garlic, minced

2 tsps white wine vinegar

1/4 cup dry white wine

6 oz. mozzarella

1/2 tsp salt

1/2 tsp black pepper

2 tsps chopped oregano

Preparation

1. Cook penne pasta according to instructions on the package.

Note: exclude oil and salt.

2. Add green beans into pasta while it cooks, at the last 3 minutes.

3. Drain pasta, retaining 1 cup cooking juices.

4. In the meantime, add olive oil into a big skillet over med-high heat.

5. Add the eggplants into the oil and stir cook for 4-5 minutes until softened.

6. Add garlic into the skillet and cook for a minute until aromatic.

7. Add 1/2 of the tomatoes and cook for 2-3 minutes until juices are just released.

8. Add the wine into the skillet and stir cook until almost all the wine is absorbed.

9. Add beans and pasta into the skillet and toss until wholly combined.

10. Slowly add the retained cooking juices from the pasta into skillet mixture.

Note: add a couple of tbsps per time.

11. Add salt, vinegar and the remaining half of the tomatoes and stir until combined.

12. Split cooked pasta between serving bowls and top with pepper, oregano and mozzarella.

Nutritional Information/Serving

Calories 428 kcal, Sodium 361mg, Carbs 56g, Protein 17g, Fat 14g

Feta Tomato Panmolle

Preparation Time: 15 minutes

Cook Time: 5 minutes

Serves: 4 servings

Ingredients

4 oz. (cut into 1" slices) French bread

2 lbs. (halved) heirloom tomatoes

1 (3 ounces) block feta cheese

1/4 cup (divided) olive oil

1/4 tsp black pepper

1/4 tsp salt

1/2 cup red onion, sliced thin

1 (14.5 ounces) can {rinsed & drained} cannellini beans, unsalted

2 tsps red wine vinegar

1/2 cup fresh chopped oregano

Preparation

1. Heat up grill to (450°F-550°F) high heat.

2. Brush the bread and tomatoes with 1 tbsp olive oil and transfer feta, bread and tomatoes onto the grates of the preheated grill.

3. Grill bread mixture for 1-2 minutes on a side, until charred.

4. Flip mixture and grill for 1-2 more minutes until charred.

5. Transfer grilled bread mixture into a platter and evenly season with pepper and salt.

6. Let sit until able to touch for 5 minutes before cutting bigger bread and tomatoes into smaller chunks.

7. Add the reserved 3 tbsps olive oil, vinegar, oregano, onion, beans, bread and tomatoes into a big bowl and toss until combined.

8. Split Tuscan salad between serving plates and top with crumbled feta.

9. Serve and enjoy.

Nutritional Information/Serving

Calories 381 kcal, Sodium 530mg, Carbs 39g, Protein 13g, Fat 21g

Turkey Zucchini Pizza

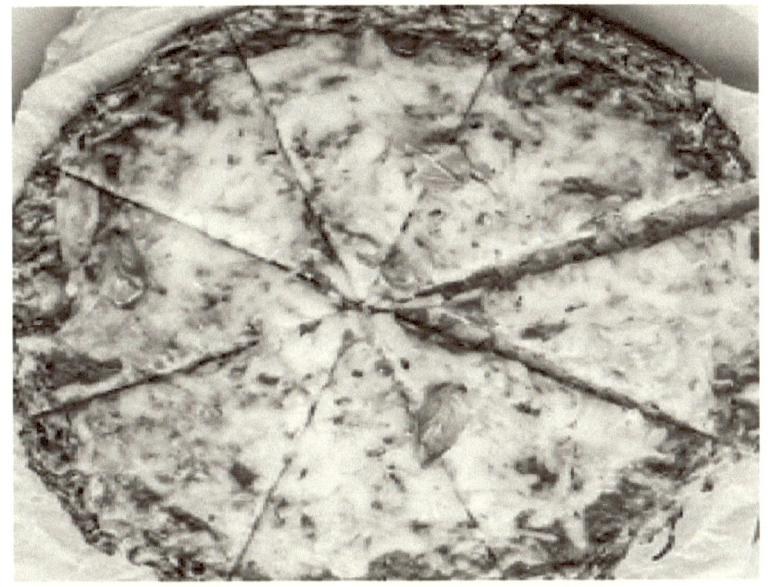

Preparation Time: 5 minutes

Cook Time: 16 minutes

Serves: 4 servings

Ingredients

1 cup zucchini, sliced thin

3 oz. mild Italian turkey sausage, ground

3 (7") pizza crusts, prebaked

1/4 cup (divided) basil pesto, frozen

1/8 tsp red pepper, crushed

3 oz. (sliced very thin) fresh mozzarella cheese

2 tbsps fresh oregano leaves

Preparation

1. Heat up oven to 450°F.

2. Place a small nonstick skillet over med-high heat.

3. Stir cook sausage in the skillet for about 4-5 minutes until well cooked.

Note: use wooden spoon to break up sausage.

4. Move cooked sausage into the platter.

5. Add 1 tbsp pesto and zucchini into the skillet and stir cook for about 3 minutes until just softened.

6. Remove skillet from heat.

7. Add the reserved 3 tbsps pesto over pizza crusts, spread evenly and transfer into a baking sheet.

8. Add red pepper, mozzarella, sausage and zucchini mixture over each crust and transfer into the preheated oven.

9. Bake for 7-8 minutes until the cheese melts and the crust edges are crispy.

10. Remove pizza from the oven and evenly sprinkle with oregano leaves.

11. Slice each pizza into 4 slices and serve at once.

Nutritional Information/Serving

Calories 392 kcal, Sodium 782mg, Carbs 44g, Protein 15g, Fat 22g

Cucumber Turkey Salad

Preparation Time: 10 minutes

Cook Time: 0 minutes

Serves: 6 servings

Ingredients

1 cup fresh baby spinach

2 cups cilantro leaves

1 tbsp pine nuts, toasted

2 tbsps fresh lime juice

1 (smashed) medium garlic clove

1 tbsp Parmesan cheese, grated

1/4 tsp black pepper

1 tsp salt

4 cups rotisserie chicken, shredded

1/2 cup olive oil

1 (15 ounces) can {drained & rinsed} chickpeas, unsalted

2 cups shelled edamame, cooked

4 cups arugula, loosely packed

1 cup English cucumber, chopped

Preparation

1. Add pepper, salt, garlic, cheese, pine nuts, lime juice, spinach and cilantro into a food processor and process for 1 minute, until a smooth consistency is reached.

2. Add olive oil into the running processor and process for a minute until a smooth consistency is reached.

3. Add cucumber, chickpeas, edamame and turkey into a big bowl and stir until combined.

4. Add pesto into the bowl and toss until combined.

5. Split 2/3 cup arugula into each six bowls, top each bowl with 1 cup turkey salad mixture.

6. Serve at once.

Nutritional Information/Serving

Calories 482 kcal, Sodium 465mg, Carbs 22g, Protein 40g, Fat 26g

Arugula Salad with Meatloaf

Preparation Time: 10 minutes

Cook Time: 10 minutes

Serves: 4 servings

Ingredients

5 oz. lean ground lamb

10 oz. sirloin, ground

1/3 cup red onion, grated

1/3 cup dry breadcrumbs

4 tsps fresh chopped basil

4 tsps fresh mint, chopped

1/4 tsp allspice, ground

3/8 tsp (divided) salt

3 minced garlic cloves

1/4 tsp red pepper, crushed

Cooking spray

1 (beaten lightly) egg, large

2 oz. crumbled feta, low-fat

1/2 cup plain Greek yogurt, no-fat

1 tbsp olive oil

2 tbsps (divided) fresh lime juice

4 cups baby arugula leaves

1/4 tsp black pepper, freshly ground

1 1/2 cups cucumber (peeled, seeded and crossways sliced into 1/4" thick slices) cucumber

Preparation

1. Heat up oven to 450°F.

2. Add breadcrumbs, ground lamb, ground sirloin, and red onion into a big bowl and combine.

3. Add the egg, minced garlic, crushed red bell pepper, allspice, salt, 3 tsps basil and 3 tsps mint into the meat mixture and combine.

4. Fill 8 cooking spray coated muffin cups with the meat mixture and press.

5. Transfer muffin cups into the preheated oven and bake for 7 minutes.

6. Broil over high heat for 3 minutes until well cooked.

7. Add 1 tsp thyme, 1 tsp mint, 1 tbsp lime juice, feta and yogurt into a food processor and process until combined.

8. Add pepper, 1/8 tsp salt, olive oil and 1 tbsp lime juice into a bowl and combine.

9. Add cucumber and arugula into the lime juice mixture and toss to combine.

Nutritional Information/Serving

Calories 347 kcal, Sodium 588mg, Carbs 13.5g, Protein 33.9g, Fat 17.3g

Creamy Turkey Marsala

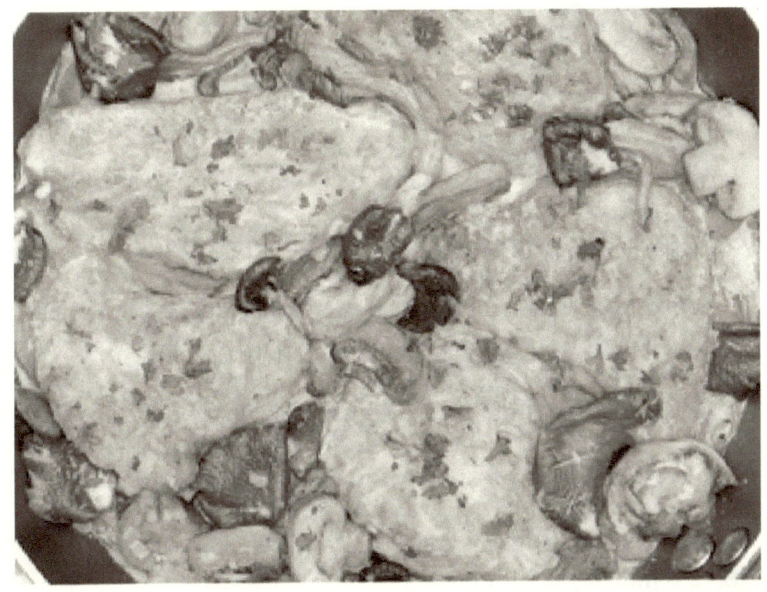

Preparation Time: 10 minutes

Cook Time: 20 minutes

Serves: 4 servings

Ingredients

4 (4 ounces) turkey breast cutlets, boneless, skinless

2 tbsps (divided) olive oil

1/2 tsp (divided) kosher salt

3/4 tsp (divided) black pepper

4 oregano sprigs

1 (8 ounces) button mushrooms, pre-sliced

2/3 cup chicken stock, unsalted

1 tbsp flour, all-purpose

2 1/2 tbsps butter, unsalted

2/3 cup Marsala wine

Preparation

1. Add 1 tbsp olive oil into a big nonstick skillet over med-high.

2. Season turkey with 1/4 tsp salt and 1/2 tsp pepper.

3. Add seasoned turkey into the heated oil and cook for 4 minutes on each side until well cooked.

4. Take out turkey from the skillet and transfer into the bowl.

5. Add the reserved 1 tbsp olive oil into the same skillet.

6. Add oregano sprigs and mushrooms into the skillet and stir cook for about 6 minutes until browned.

7. Sprinkle flour over mushroom mixture and stir cook for a minute.

8. Add the wine and stock into the skillet and bring to boiling.

9. Cook for 2-3 more minutes until just thickened.

10. Take skillet off heat.

11. Add the butter, the reserved 1/4 tsp salt and the 1/4 tsp pepper into the skillet and stir to combine.

12. Add turkey into the skillet mixture, stir until wholly coated.

13. Get rid of the oregano sprigs before you serve.

14. Serve and enjoy.

Nutritional Information/Serving

Calories 344 kcal, Carbs 9g, Protein 28g, Fat 17g, Sodium 567mg

Veggie Lamb Meatballs with Greens

Preparation Time: 10 minutes

Cook Time: 12 minutes

Serves: 4 servings

Ingredients

1/2 cup bulgur, uncooked

1 (8 ounces) beets, cooked

3/4 tsp (divided) kosher salt

1 tsp cumin, ground

6 oz. lamb, ground

3/4 tsp black pepper, freshly ground

1 tbsp olive oil

1/3 cup almond flour

1/2 cup sour cream, reduced-fat

1/2 cup cucumber, grated

2 tbsps fresh lime juice

2 tbsps fresh mint, sliced thin

4 cups mixed baby greens

Preparation

1. Heat up oven to 425°F.

2. Add beets into a food processor and process until chopped finely.

3. Add almond flour, ground lamb, pepper, 1/2 tsp salt, cumin, bulgur and beets into a bowl, combine and form into 12 balls.

4. Add olive oil into a big oven secure skillet over med-high heat.

5. Add meatballs into the heated oil and cook until evenly browned, for about 4 minutes.

6. Transfer skillet with browned meatballs into the preheated oven and bake until well cooked, for 8 minutes.

7. Add lime juice, mint, sour cream, cucumber and 1/4 tsp salt into a small bowl and combine.

8. Split mixed baby greens between four plates, topped with cucumber mixture and meatballs.

Nutritional Information/Serving

Calories 338 kcal, Sodium 458mg, Carbs 25g, Protein 14g, Fat 21g

Mediterranean Shrimp Spaghetti

Preparation Time: 10 minutes

Cook Time: 20 minutes

Serves: 4 servings

Ingredients

1 lb. raw medium shrimp, peeled and deveined

8 oz. whole-grain spaghetti, uncooked

3/4 tsp (divided) salt

1/2 tsp black pepper

2 cups leek, chopped

1 1/2 tbsps (divided) olive oil

2 cups baby sweet peas, frozen and thawed

1 tbsp garlic, chopped

2 tsps lime zest

1/4 cup heavy cream

2 tbsps fresh dill, chopped

2 tbsps fresh lime juice

Preparation

1. Cook pasta according instructions on the package.

Note: exclude oil and salt.

2. Retain 1/2 cup cooking juices from the cooked pasta and let pasta sit to keep warm.

3. In the meantime, use paper towel to pat dry shrimp and sprinkle with 1/4 tsp salt and pepper until wholly coated.

4. Add 1/2 of the olive oil into the big nonstick skillet over high heat.

5. Add the seasoned shrimp into the heated oil and stir cook for 3-4 minutes until well cooked.

6. Plate cooked shrimp, place lid over plate to keep warm.

7. Adjust heat to med-high, add 1/2 tsp salt, the remaining oil, garlic and leek into the skillet and stir cook for 2-3 minutes until the leek is just soft.

8. Add the reserved cooking juice, lime juice, lime zest, cream and peas into the skillet mixture and adjust to med-heat.

9. Simmer the mixture for 2-3 minutes until sauce is just thickened.

10. Add shrimp into the sauce and toss until wholly coated.

11. Split pasta between serving bowls and top with dill, sauce and shrimp.

12. Serve and enjoy.

Nutritional Information/Serving

Calories 446 kcal, Sodium 649 kcal, Carbs 59g, Protein 28g, Fat 13g

Creamy Mediterranean Hummus

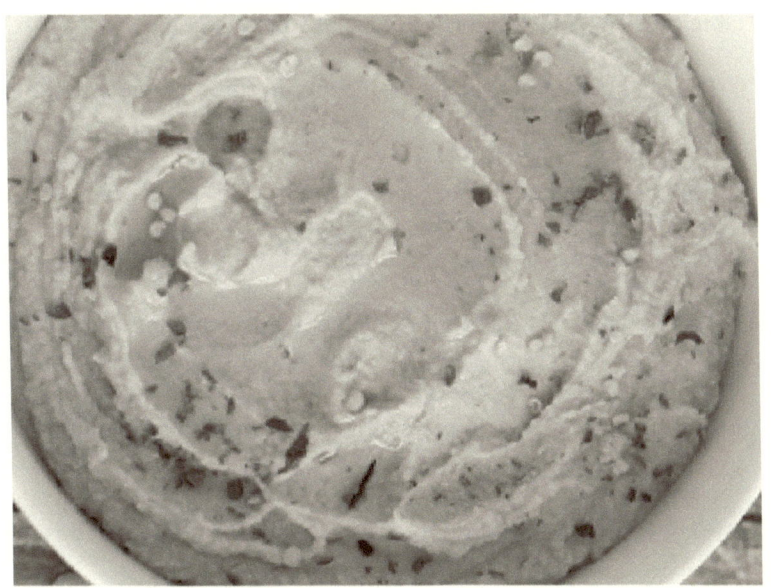

Preparation Time: 15 minutes

Cook Time: 20 minutes

Serves: 8 servings

Ingredients

1-2 minced garlic cloves

3 cups cooked chickpeas

1/3 cup tahini paste

3-4 ice cubes

1 lime, juiced

½ teaspoon kosher salt

Olive oil

Preparation

1. Add 1 1/2 teaspoon baking soda and cooked or canned chickpeas into a big bowl with just enough hot water to cover.

2. Place a handful of chickpeas under cold running water and rub until skins are peeled.

3. Transfer peeled chickpeas into a bowl.

4. Repeat process until no unpeeled chickpea remains.

5. Add minced garlic and the peeled chickpeas into a food processor bowl and process until a powdery and smooth consistency is reached.

6. Add lime juice, salt, tahini and ice cubes into the running processor with the chickpea mixture.

7. Process mixture for 4 minutes until a smooth consistency is reached.

Tip: if mixture is too thick, gradually add hot water into running processor until fully incorporated and thinned out.

8. Scoop and spread hummus into serving bowls and top with a liberal dribble of olive oil.

9. Enjoy with desired veggies and warm pita.

Nutritional Information/Serving

Calories 176 kcal, Protein 7.2g, Total Carbs 19.4g, Sodium 153.2mg, Total Fat 8.7g

Veggie Tagine

Preparation Time: 15 minutes

Cook Time: 40 minutes

Serves: 4 servings

Ingredients

2 (peeled and chopped) medium yellow onions

1/4 cup olive oil

2 (peeled and chopped) big carrots

8–10 (peeled and chopped) garlic cloves

1 (peeled and cubed) big sweet potato

2 (peeled and cubed) big russet potatoes

1 tablespoon Harissa spice blend

Salt

1 teaspoon cinnamon, ground

1 teaspoon coriander, ground

2 cups canned whole peeled tomatoes

1/2 teaspoon turmeric, ground

1 qt. veggie broth, reduced sodium

1/2 generous cup dried apricot, chopped

1 lime, juiced

2 cups chickpeas, cooked

1 handful fresh cilantro leaves

Preparation

1. Add olive oil into a big heavy pot over med-heat.

2. Heat oil until it shimmers.

3. Adjust heat to med-high and add onions into the hot oil and stir-saute for 5 minutes.

4. Add the chopped vegetables and garlic into the pot, sprinkle with spices and salt and toss until to combined.

5. Stir cook veggie mixture for 5-7 minutes.

Tip: Stir often with a wooden spoon.

6. Add the broth, apricot and tomatoes into the pot and sprinkle with a pinch of salt.

7. Cook mixture for 10 minutes on med-high heat.

8. Adjust heat to low heat, place lid over pot and simmer until vegetables are softened, for 20-25 more minutes.

9. Add chickpeas into the veggie mixture, stir to combine and cook over low heat for 5 extra minutes.

10. Add fresh cilantro leaves and lime juice into the mixture.

11. Check for seasoning and adjust as necessary.

12. Split tagine into serving bowls and dribble liberally with olive oil.

13. Serve with brown rice or crusty bread.

Nutritional Information/Serving

Calories 448 kcal, Protein 16.9g, Total Carbs 60.7g, Sodium 405.4mg, Total Fat 18.4g

Oregano Watermelon Salad

Preparation Time: 10 minutes

Cook Time: 0 minutes

Serves: 4 servings

Ingredients (dressing)

2 tablespoons lemon juice

2 tablespoons honey

1 pinch salt

1 tablespoon olive oil

Salad

1 (cubed) English cucumber

1 (5 pound) {peeled and cubed} watermelon

15 (torn) fresh oregano leaves

15 (torn) fresh mint leaves

1/2 cup feta cheese, crumbled

Preparation

1. Add every dressing ingredient into a small bowl, whisk until combined and let sit until needed.

2. Add fresh herbs, cucumbers and water into a big bowl and combine.

3. Empty dressing mixture over salad and toss lightly until combined.

4. Serve garnished with feta cheese.

Nutritional Information/Serving

Calories 295 kcal, Protein 6.3g, Total Carbs 55.9g, Sodium 761.4mg, Total Fat 8.4g

Olive Feta Pasta

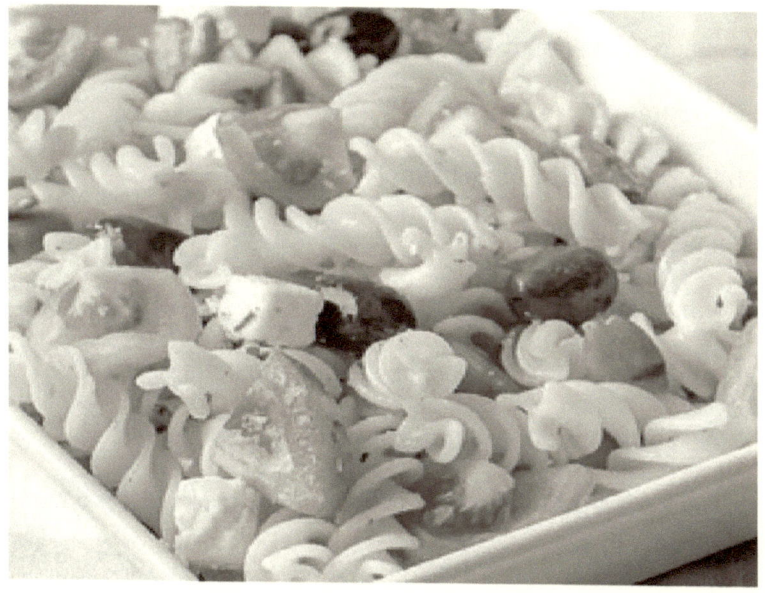

Preparation Time: 10 minutes

Cook Time: 10 minutes

Serves: 6 servings

Ingredients

1/2 cup olive oil

1 pound thin spaghetti

Salt

4 crushed garlic cloves

12 ounces halved grape tomatoes

1 cup fresh cilantro, chopped

1 teaspoon black pepper

3 (trim top and chop green and white parts) scallions

1/4 cup (pitted and halved) olives

6 ounces (drained) marinated artichoke hearts

10–15 (torn) fresh oregano

1/4 cup feta cheese, crumbled

1 lime, zested

Preparation

1. Add enough water into a pot and bring to boiling.

2. Add little olive oil, salt and pasta into the boiling water.

3. Cook pasta according to directions on the package, for 6 minutes or more until al dente.

4. Add 1/2 cup olive oil into a big cast iron skillet over med-heat and heat.

5. Adjust heat to low heat and add a pinch of salt and garlic into the oil.

6. Stir cook garlic for 10 seconds.

7. Add chopped scallions, tomatoes and parsley into the skillet mixture, stir and cook for 30 seconds until warmed through over low heat.

8. Remove cooked spaghetti from heat and drain the water.

9. Pour the warm garlic/olive oil sauce into the drained pasta and toss until evenly coated.

10. Add black pepper into the pasta mixture and toss until evenly combined.

11. Add every other ingredient into the pasta mixture, toss again and serve into serving bowls.

12. Serve topped with feta and chopped oregano.

Nutritional Information/Serving

Calories 389 kcal, Protein 10.7g, Total Carbs 51.1g, Total Fat 16.6g

Turkey Shawarma

Preparation Time: 10 minutes

Cook Time: 30 minutes

Serves: 6 servings

Ingredients

3/4 tablespoon turmeric powder

3/4 tablespoon cumin, ground

3/4 tablespoon garlic powder

3/4 tablespoon coriander, ground

1/2 teaspoon cloves, ground

3/4 tablespoon paprika

Salt

1/2 teaspoon cayenne pepper

1 (sliced thin) large onion

8 turkey thighs, skinless, boneless

1/3 cup olive oil

1 big lime, juiced

Serve with

Greek Tzatziki sauce

6 pita pockets

Baby arugula

Mediterranean salad

Preparation

1. Add cloves, sweet paprika, garlic powder, coriander, turmeric and cumin into a small bowl, combine well and let sit until needed.

2. Pat dry turkey thighs and sprinkle with salt until wholly seasoned on all sides.

3. Slice turkey into small chunks and transfer into a big bowl.

4. Add cumin mixture over turkey and toss until evenly covered.

5. Add olive oil, lime juice and onions into the turkey mixture and toss once more to combine.

6. Place lid over turkey bowl and transfer into a refrigerator for 3 hours or more until turkey is marinated.

7. Heat up oven to 425°F and grease a baking pan lightly.

8. Remove turkey from the refrigerator and let sit for some minutes until cooled.

9. Add onions and marinated turkey onto the prepared baking pan and spread in a single layer.

10. Transfer baking sheet into the preheated oven and bake for 30 minutes until roasted.

11. In the meantime, prepare Tzatziki sauce as desired and prepare the pita pockets.

12. Open up pita pockets and spread with Tzatziki sauce.

13. Add Mediterranean salad, arugula and turkey shawarma into the opened pocket, close pockets and serve at once.

Nutritional Information/Serving

Calories 227 kcal, Protein 4.7g, Total Carbs 22.5g, Total Fat 14.8g

Yummy Greek Tzatziki Sauce

Preparation Time: 15 minutes

Cook Time: 0 minutes

Serves: 12 (2-3 tablespoons) servings

Ingredients

1 teaspoon (divided) kosher salt

3/4 (peel partially and sliced) English cucumber

1 teaspoon white vinegar

4-5 (peeled and minced) garlic cloves

2 cups Greek yogurt

1 tablespoon olive oil

1/4 teaspoon white pepper, ground

Serve with

Veggies, sliced

Pita bread, warmed

Preparation

1. Add peeled and sliced cucumbers into a food processor and process until evenly grated.

2. Season grated cucumbers with 1/2 teaspoon salt and toss until coated.

3. Pour salted cucumbers into a fine mesh strainer and strain over a deep bowl.

4. Squeeze the drained cucumber in a cheese cloth until no liquid remain and let sit.

5. Add olive, white vinegar, 1/2 teaspoon salt and garlic into a big bowl and mix until well combined.

6. Add the squeezed cucumber into olive oil mixture.

7. Add white pepper and Greek yogurt into the olive oil mixture and stir until combine.

8. Place lid over mixture until well covered and transfer into a refrigerator for some hours.

9. Stir sauce before serving, and scoop into serving bowls, topped with olive oil.

10. Serve with sliced veggies and warmed pita bread.

Nutritional Information/Serving

Calories 34 kcal, Protein 0.1g, Total Carbs 0.5g, Total Fat 1.2g

Veggies with Baked Halibut

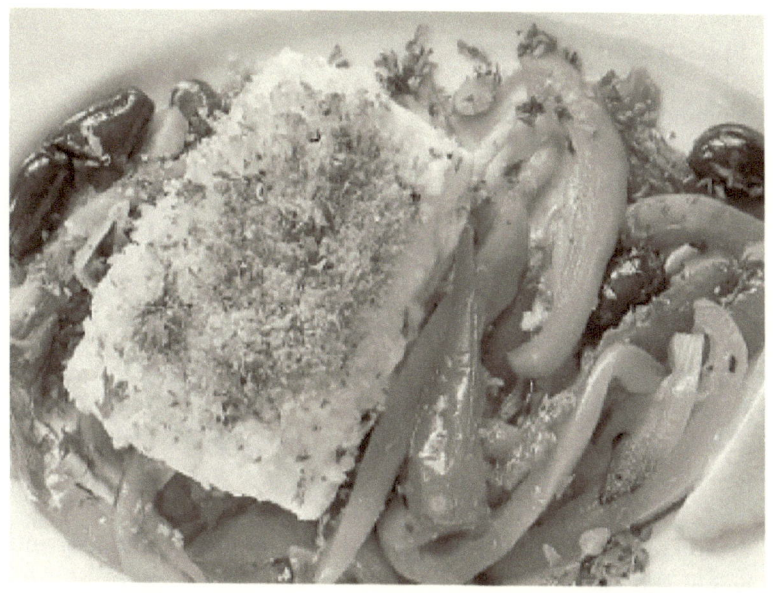

Preparation Time: 10 minutes

Cook Time: 15 minutes

Serves: 6 servings

Ingredients (sauce)

1 cup olive oil

2 lime, zested and juiced

2 teaspoons dill weed

1 1/2 tablespoons garlic, freshly minced

1/2 teaspoon black pepper, ground

1 teaspoon salt

1/2-3/4 teaspoon coriander, ground

1 teaspoon basil, dried

Baked Halibut

1 pound cherry tomatoes

1 pound fresh green beans

1 1/2 pounds (slice into 1 1/2" pieces) halibut fillet

1 (sliced into half moons) large yellow onion

Preparation

1. Heat up oven to 425°F.

2. Add every sauce ingredient into a big bowl and whisk until well combined.

3. Add onions, tomatoes and green beans into sauce and toss until wholly combined.

4. Transfer the veggies into a big baking sheet using a big slotted spoon.

5. Move the veggies to the side of the baking sheet and spread in a single layer.

6. Transfer the fish fillet into the sauce and toss until wholly coated.

7. Transfer the coated fillets onto the other side of the baking sheet.

8. Empty the remaining sauce over the veggies and fish fillets.

9. Season the baking sheet mixture with a little salt until lightly seasoned.

10. Transfer baking sheet into the preheated oven and bake for 10 minutes.

11. Move baking sheet to the broiler and broil until the cherry tomatoes starts to pop, for 3 more minutes.

Note: Make sure you do not burn the fish.

12. Serve veggies and baked halibut with favorite pasta or grain.

Nutritional Information/Serving

Calories 649 kcal, Protein 31.8g, Total Carbs 57.3g, Total Fat 32.9g

Grilled Turkey Souvlaki

Preparation Time: 20 minutes

Cook Time: 15 minutes

Serves: 12 servings

Ingredients (marinade)

2 tablespoons basil, dried

10 peeled garlic cloves

1 teaspoon sweet paprika

1 teaspoon dried thyme

1 teaspoon black pepper

1 teaspoon Kosher salt

1/4 cup dry white wine

1/4 cup olive oil

2 bay leaves

1 lime, juiced

Turkey

2 1/2 pounds (remove fat and cut into 1 1/2" pieces) turkey breast, skinless boneless

Pita

Tzatziki sauce

Greek pita bread

Cucumber, sliced

Tomato, sliced

Kalamata olives

Onions, sliced

Preparation

1. Add every marinade ingredient excluding the bay leaves into a small food processor bowl and process until combined.

2. Add bay leaves and turkey into a big bowl and empty the marinade mixture over turkey.

3. Toss turkey mixture until evenly coated.

4. Place lid over turkey mixture and transfer into a refrigerator for 2 hours or more until marinated.

5. Place 12 bamboo skewers in water for 30-45 minutes until well soaked.

6. In the meantime, prepare the veggies, tzatziki sauce and the pita bread.

7. Thread the marinated turkey chunks through the soaked skewers.

8. Heat up an outdoor grill to med-high heat and grease grates lightly.

9. Working in batches, transfer the skewers onto the preheated grill and cook until an internal temperature of 155° is reached, for 5 minutes on every side.

TIP: Lightly baste turkey skewers with remaining marinade and turn skewers to ensure even browning.

10. Move browned turkey skewers to a plate and let sit for 3 minutes to cool.

11. Repeat process until no turkey remains.

12. Grill pitas lightly until warmed.

13. Remove turkey from skewers and get rid of the skewers.

14. Spread tzatziki sauce over pita as desired.

15. Add turkey chunks, olives and vegetables on pita and serve.

Nutritional Information/Serving

Calories 168 kcal, Protein 22g, Total Carbs 1.8g, Total Fat 7.7g

DINNER

Grapefruit Lamb Chops

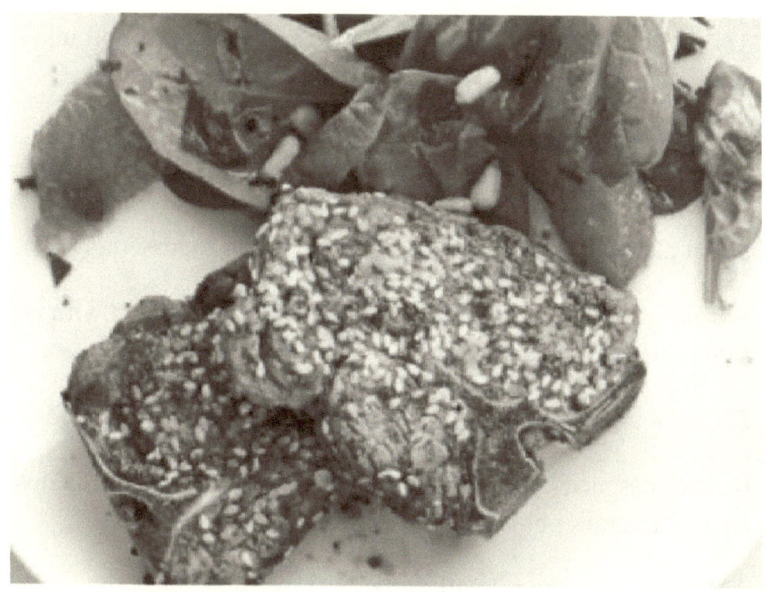

Preparation Time: 10 minutes

Cook Time: 9 minutes

Serves: 4 servings

Ingredients

2 tsps grapefruit rind, grated

4 tsps (divided) olive oil

8 (4 oz.) {trimmed} lamb rib chops

1 tbsp grapefruit juice

1/2 tsp black pepper, freshly ground

1 tsp salt

3 tbsps balsamic vinegar

Cooking spray

Preparation

1. Add grapefruit juice, grapefruit rind and 1 tbsp olive oil into a big plastic bag.

2. Add lamb into the mixture in the plastic bag, seal the lid and shake until wholly coated.

3. Let plastic bag mixture sit for 10 minutes at room temp.

4. Take out the marinated lamb from the bag and season with pepper and salt until evenly covered.

5. Coat a big grill pan with cooking spray and place over med-high heat.

6. Add seasoned lamb into the grill pan and cook until well cooked, for about 2 minutes per side.

7. Add vinegar into a small skillet over med-high heat and bring to boiling.

8. Cook vinegar until syrupy for 3 more minutes.

9. Dribble the remaining 1 tsp olive oil and the vinegar syrup over the lamb and serve.

Nutritional Information/Serving

Calories 593 kcal, Carbs 3g, Fat 43g, Protein 43g, Sodium 720mg

Veggie Parmesan Pizza

Preparation Time: 10 minutes

Cook Time: 11 minutes

Serves: 4 servings

Ingredients

1 tbsp cornmeal

Cooking spray

2 tbsps pesto, store-bought

1 (13.8 oz.) can pizza crust dough, chilled

1 (9 oz.) {thawed, drained and chop roughly} artichoke hearts, frozen

1/2 cup part-skim mozzarella cheese, shredded

2 tbsps Parmesan cheese, shredded

1 oz. prosciutto, sliced thin

1 1/2 tbsps lime juice

1 1/2 cups arugula leaves

Preparation

1. Heat up oven to 500°F and set rack in the last position.

2. Use cooking spray to evenly cover a baking sheet.

3. Scatter corn meal over sprayed baking dish.

4. Add pizza crust dough into the baking sheet and form into a 14-by-10" frame.

5. Add pesto over crust, spread evenly and leave a 1/2" limit.

6. Scatter mozzarella cheese over pizza crust dough before transferring onto the prepared rack in the preheated oven.

7. Bake pizza for 5 minutes and remove pizza from the oven.

8. Scatter parmesan, prosciutto slices and chopped artichokes over pizza top.

9. Place back pizza into the last rack of the oven and bake for 6 more minutes until crust is browned.

10. Add arugula into a bowl and dribble in the lime juice evenly.

11. Toss arugula lightly until combined.

12. Add the arugula over pizza and slice as desired into 8 wedges.

Nutritional Information/Serving

Calories 435 kcal, Carbs 52g, Fat 10g, Protein 33g, Sodium 664mg

Cheesy Olive Rigatoni Pasta

Preparation Time: 10 minutes

Cook Time: 10 minutes

Serves: 6 servings

Ingredients

1 1/4 cups green olives, pitted

1 lb. rigatoni, uncooked

1/2 cup cilantro leaves

1/2 cup toasted sliced almonds

1 garlic clove, large

1/4 tsp black pepper, freshly ground

1 tsp white wine vinegar

2 tbsps water

1/2 cup Romano cheese, grated

Preparation

1. Cook rigatoni pasta according to instructions on the package until al dente.

Note: Exclude oil and salt.

2. Drain rigatoni pasta and keep 6 tbsps of the pasta's cooking juices.

3. Add garlic, black pepper, cilantro, toasted sliced almond and olives into a food process and process until mixture is roughly chopped.

4. Add 1 tsp vinegar and 2 tbsps water through the opening at the top while the processor is running.

5. Process until a finely chopped consistency is reached.

6. Add olive mixture, the retained 4 tbsps cooking juices and pasta into a big bowl and toss until combined.

7. Slowly add 2 tbsps cooking juices into the pasta mixture until desired consistency is reached, toss mixture until well coated.

8. Serve and top with grated Romano cheese.

Nutritional Information/Serving

Calories 493 kcal, Carbs 65g, Fat 17g, Protein 15g, Sodium 468mg

Rice with Lamb kofta

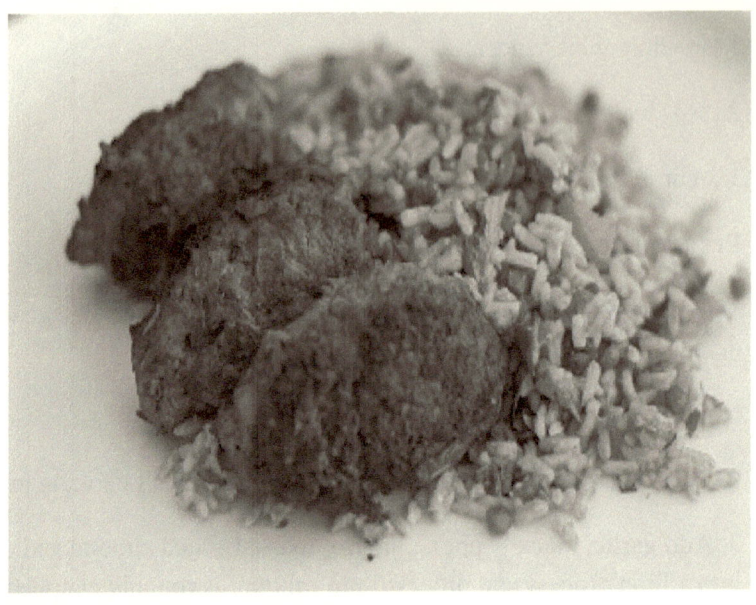

Preparation Time: 10 minutes

Cook Time: 20 minutes

Serves: 4 servings

Ingredients (rice)

1 tsp saffron threads

1 (3.5 oz.) bag jasmine rice (boil-in-bag)

2 tbsps green onions, sliced thin

Kofta

2 tbsps onion, grated

2 tbsps parsley, minced

1 tsp cumin, ground

2 tbsps plain Greek yogurt

1 tsp turmeric

1 tsp coriander, ground

1/2 tsp salt

2 tsps garlic, minced

1 lb. lean ground lamb

1/4 tsp black pepper

Cooking spray

Sauce

1/4 cup roasted red bell pepper, chopped

1/2 cup plain Greek yogurt

1 tsp coriander, ground

1 tsp cumin, ground

1/2 tsp red pepper, crushed

2 tsps garlic, minced

1/4 tsp salt

Preparation

1. Add saffron and jasmine rice bag into boiling water and cook according to instructions on the package.

2. Drain water and use a fork to fluff the cooked rice.

3. Sprinkle green onions over fluffed rice.

4. In the meantime, add ground lamb, black pepper, salt, minced garlic, turmeric, coriander, cumin, yogurt, onion and parsley into a bowl and combine.

5. Form lamb mixture into 12 oval patties.

6. Coat a big nonstick skillet with cooking spray and place over med-high heat.

7. Add patties into the heated pan and cook until well cooked on every side, for 10 minutes.

8. In the meantime, add every other ingredient including the 1/2 cup yogurt into a bowl and combine.

9. Serve rice, sauce and kofta.

Nutritional Information/Serving

Calories 364 kcal, Carbs 39g, Fat 12g, Protein 33g, Sodium 534mg

Greek Roasted Potatoes

Preparation Time: 15 minutes

Cook Time: 50 minutes

Serves: 6 servings

Ingredients (seasoning mix)

1 teaspoon black pepper

1 teaspoon salt, seasoned

1 teaspoon fresh basil

1 teaspoon sweet paprika

Potatoes

8 (chopped) big garlic cloves

4 (peeled, washed and sliced into wedges) big baking potatoes

1 lime, juiced

4 tablespoons olive oil

1/2 cup Parmesan cheese, grated

1 1/4 cup broth

1 cup (coarsely chopped) cilantro leaves

Preparation

1. Heat up oven to 400°F.

2. Lightly oil a big baking dish.

3. Add seasoning mix into a small, combine well and let sit until needed.

4. Add potato wedges into the prepared baking dish and sprinkle with the seasoning mix.

5. Toss potato mixture until wholly coated.

6. Add broth, lime juice, olive oil and chopped garlic into a bowl and whisk until combined.

7. Empty broth mixture over potatoes.

8. Place foil over baking dish until covered and transfer into the preheated oven.

9. Roast potatoes for 40 minutes.

10. Remove foil from the baking dish and top with the parmesan cheese.

11. Return baking dish into the oven and roast until a little crust begins to form, potatoes are well cooked and nice golden brown, for 10-15 more minutes.

12. Serve garnished with fresh chopped cilantro.

Nutritional Information/Serving

Calories 409 kcal, Protein 13.8g, Total Carbs 77g, Sodium 434.9mg, Total Fat 8.2g

Colorful Veggie Bowl with Dressing

Preparation Time: 15 minutes

Cook Time: 10 minutes

Serves: 4 servings

Ingredients

1/2 cup bulgur, uncooked

1 cup water, boiling

1 1/2 tbsps olive oil

2 (15 ounces) cans (washed and drained) chickpeas, unsalted

4 cups kale, chopped

2 cups carrots, finely chopped

1/2 cup fresh cilantro leaves

1/2 cup (sliced straight up) shallots

1/2 tsp black pepper

3/4 tsp (divided) kosher salt

2 tbsps olive oil

1/2 (peeled and pitted) avocado

1 tbsp water

1 tbsp fresh lime juice

1 garlic clove

1 tbsp tahini

1/4 tsp turmeric, ground

Preparation

1. Add bulgur and the boiling water into an average bowl, combine and let sit for 10 minutes before draining.

2. Add olive oil into a big skillet over high heat.

3. Add the carrots and the pat dried chickpeas into the heated oil, stir cook for about 6 minutes until chickpeas is browned.

4. Add the kale into the skillet, place lid over skillet and cook for about 2 minutes until the carrots are softened and kale is just wilted.

5. Add pepper, 1/2 tsp salt, cilantro, shallots and chickpea mixture into the bulgur bowl and toss until combined.

6. Add 1/4 tsp salt, turmeric, garlic, tahini, 1 tbsp water, lime juice, 2 tablespoons and avocado into a food processor and process until a smooth consistency is reached.

7. Split into 4 serving bowls and dribble with avocado dressing, serve and enjoy.

Nutritional Information/Serving

Calories 520 kcal, Carbs 68g, Protein 18g, Fat 20g, Sodium 495mg

Broccoli Panko Salmon

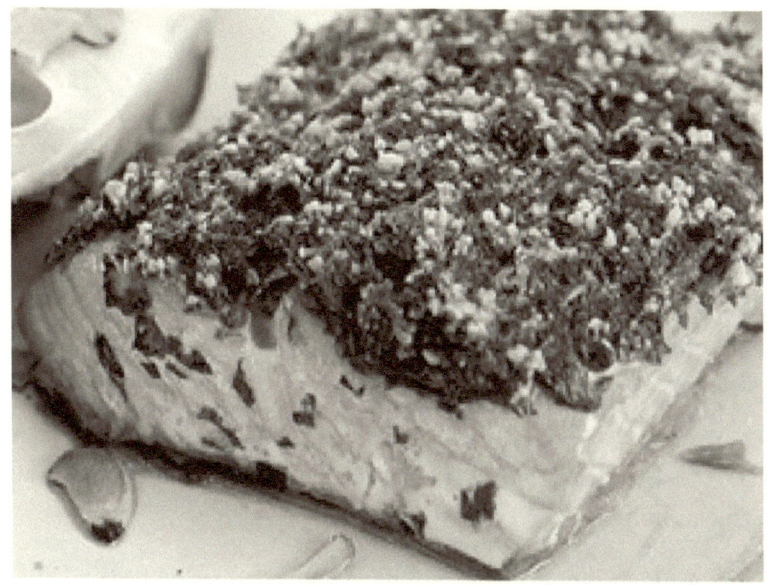

Preparation Time: 10 minutes

Cook Time: 15 minutes

Serves: 4 servings

Ingredients

1 1/2 tbsps mayo

1 1/2 tbsps Dijon mustard

1/2 tsp (divided) black pepper

3/4 tsp (divided) salt

1/2 cup panko, whole-wheat

4 (6 ounces) salmon fillets, skinless

2 tsps (divided) lime rind, grated

1 tbsp (divided)fresh tarragon, chopped

2 1/2 cups (trimmed) broccoli florets

2 tbsps (divided) olive oil

2 tsps fresh lime juice

1/3 cup shallots, sliced thin

Preparation

1. Add 1/4 tsp pepper, 1/2 tsp salt, mayo and mustard into a flat-bottomed bowl and combine.

2. Scoop mixture over salmon fillets until evenly coated.

3. Add 1 tsp lime rind, 1 1/2 tsps tarragon and panko crumbs into a bowl and combine.

4. Sprinkle salmon fillets with the panko mixture and press until it sticks.

5. Add 1 tablespoon olive oil into a big nonstick skillet over med-heat.

6. Cautiously add the salmon fillets into the oil with the breaded side down.

7. Cook until fillets are golden, for 3-4 minutes.

8. Flip fillets and cook until cooked to desire, for 3-4 more minutes.

9. Take fillets out of the skillet, place in a plate and cover to keep warm.

10. Adjust to med-high heat.

11. Add the reserved olive oil into the skillet and add the shallots and broccoli florets.

12. Stir cook veggies for about 3 minutes.

13. Add the lime juice, the remaining lime rind, the remaining tarragon, the remaining pepper and the remaining salt into the skillet and cook until broccoli florets are crisp-soft, for 2 minutes.

14. Serve and enjoy.

Nutritional Information/Serving

Calories 387 kcal, Sodium 630mg, Carbs 13g, Protein 39g, Fat 18g

Grilled Salmon with Veggie Salsa

Preparation Time: 15 minutes

Cook Time: 6 minutes

Serves: 4 servings

Ingredients

1 cup cherry tomatoes, halved

2 cups avocado, peeled, pitted and cubed

1/2 tsp serrano chile, chopped

2 tbsps fresh chopped parsley

1 tsp fresh lemon juice

1 1/2 tbsps shallot, sliced

3/4 tsp (divided) black pepper

1 tsp (divided) salt

4 (6 ounces ea) salmon fillets, skin-on

1 tbsp olive oil

Preparation

1. Heat up grill to (450°F) med-high heat.

2. Add shallot, serrano, parsley, tomatoes and cubed avocado into a big bowl and combine.

3. Add 1/4 tsp pepper, 1/4 tsp salt and lemon juice into a separate bowl and whisk until combined.

4. Dribble lemon juice dressing over avocado mixture and stir until wholly combined.

5. Coat salmon with olive oil on both sides and season with 1/2 tsp pepper and 3/4 tsp salt.

6. Transfer salmon onto the grill with the skin side down and cook for 3 minutes.

7. Flip salmon and cook until well cooked and opaque for 3 more minutes.

8. Serve cooked salmon with salsa and enjoy.

Nutritional Information/Serving

Calories 408 kcal, Sodium 574mg, Carbs 9g, Protein 38g, Fat 24g

Mediterranean Potatoes with Lamb

Preparation Time: 25 minutes

Cook Time: 1 hour 10 minutes

Serves: 6 servings

Ingredients

Salt and pepper

1 (5 pound) {bone-in with excess fat trimmed} leg of lamb

5 (peeled and sliced) garlic cloves

Olive oil

8 (peeled and cut into wedges) gold potatoes, medium

2 cups water

1 teaspoon paprika

1 (peeled and cut into wedges) yellow onion, medium

Fresh chopped cilantro

1 teaspoon garlic powder

Rub

2 tablespoons basil, dried

15 peeled garlic cloves

1 tablespoon paprika

2 tablespoons mint flakes, dried

1/2 cup olive oil

1/2 tablespoon nutmeg, ground

2 limes, juiced

Preparation

1. Take out meat from the fridge and let sit for 1 hour until thawed at room temperature.

2. Add every rub ingredient into a food processor, mix and process until a smooth consistency is reached.

3. Pat dry lamb and score lamb on both sides with a sharp knife.

4. Sprinkle pepper and salt over scored lamb until evenly seasoned.

5. Set oven to broil.

6. Transfer seasoned leg of lamb onto a wire rack and transfer into the oven over the highest oven rack.

7. Broil leg of lamb until finely seared on both sides for 5-7 minutes per side.

8. Take off leg of lamb from the oven, let sit to cool and set oven temperature to 375°F.

9. Slot in slices of garlic into the holes earlier made on the meat.

10. Brush meat with the wet rub on evenly coated.

11. Transfer the leg of lamb into the center of inside rack fitted roasting pan.

12. Pour 2 cups water into the base of the roasting pan.

13. Sprinkle a pinch of salt, garlic powder and paprika over onion and potato wedges and transfer the seasoned wedges to both sides of the lamb.

14. Place a big aluminum foil piece over roasting pan until covered and transfer into the center rack of the preheated oven.

15. Roast potatoes, onions and lamb for 1 hour.

16. Remove roasting plan to get rid of foil, return into the oven and cook lamb until an internal temperature of 140°F, for 10-15 more minutes.

17. Let meat rest for 20 minutes to cool before you serve.

18. Serve as desired

Nutritional Information/Serving

Calories 1060 kcal, Carbs 52g, Fat 53g, Protein 100g, Sodium 203mg

Velvety Braised Eggplant

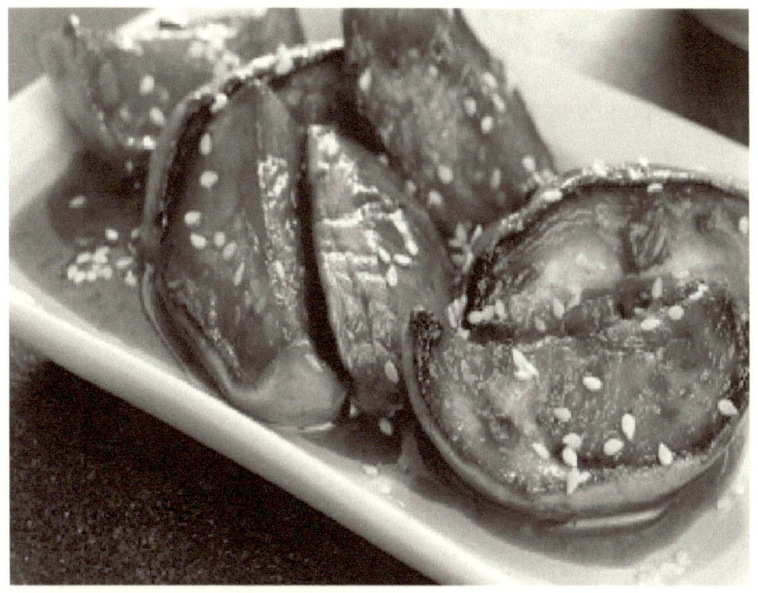

Preparation Time: 20 minutes

Cook Time: 55 minutes

Serves: 6 servings

Ingredients

Salt

1 1/2 pounds (cubed) eggplant

1 (chopped) yellow onion, big

Olive oil

1 (chopped) carrot

1 (remove insides and stems, and dice) green bell pepper

2 dry bay leaves

6 minced garlic cloves, large

1 teaspoon coriander, ground

1-1 1/2 teaspoons sweet paprika

3/4 teaspoon cinnamon, ground

1 teaspoon dry basil

1/2 teaspoon black pepper

1/2 teaspoon turmeric, ground

2 (15 ounces) cans chickpeas, retain juices in the can

1 (28 ounces) can chopped tomato

Garnish with

Fresh chopped cilantro

Preparation

1. Heat up oven to 400°F.

2. Place colander over a big bowl and add cubed eggplants.

3. Season the cubed eggplants with salt and let sit for 20 minutes.

4. Rinse eggplant cubes and pat dry.

5. Add 1/4 cup olive oil into a big brazier over med-high heat.

6. Heat oil until it shimmers.

Note: don't over heat, oil should not be smoky.

7. Add chopped carrot, peppers and onions into the oil and stir cook for 2-3 minutes.

8. Add a pinch salt, spices, bay leaf and garlic into the brazier and stir cook until aromatic for 1 more minute.

9. Add the reserved chickpea juices, chickpeas, chopped tomato and eggplant into the pot and mix well until combined.

10. Bring mixture to a roiling boil for about 10 minutes, stirring every now and then.

11. Take mixture off heat, place lid over pot and move into the preheated oven.

12. Cook eggplants until softened and well cooked, for 45 minutes.

Note: Check every now and then to see if cooking juices is drying up, add 1/2 cup water per time and stir until incorporated.

13. Take out the cooked eggplants from the oven, serve garnished with fresh chopped cilantro and dribble liberally with olive oil.

Nutritional Information/Serving

Calories 438 kcal, Protein 19g, Total Carbs 86g Sodium 248.2mg, Total Fat 5.8g

Cheesy Turkey Couscous

Preparation Time: 8 minutes

Cook Time: 12 minutes

Serves: 6 servings

Ingredients

1/2 cup tomatoes, sun-dried

2 1/3 cups (divided) water

1 3/4 cups couscous, uncooked

1 (14.5 oz.) can veggie broth

1/2 cup feta cheese, crumbled

3 cups (cooked and chopped) turkey breast

2 (6 oz.) jars (undrained) marinated artichoke hearts

1 cup fresh chopped cilantro

1/4 tsp black pepper, freshly ground

Preparation

1. Add tomatoes and 2 cups water into an oven secure bowl and combine.

2. Place bowl in a microwave oven and bring to boiling, for 3 minutes on high.

3. Place lid over bowl and let tomatoes sit until softened for 10 minutes.

4. Drain water and reserve tomatoes until needed.

5. Add veggie broth and 1/3 cup water into a big saucepan and bring to boiling.

6. Add couscous into the broth mixture and stir to combine.

7. Place lid over saucepan, adjust heat to low and simmer until softened for 8 minutes.

8. Take off saucepan from heat, add the tomatoes and every other ingredient and stir until evenly distributed.

9. Serve and enjoy.

Nutritional Information/Serving

Calories 631 kcal, Carbs 75g, Fat 15g, Protein 50g, Sodium 316mg

Turkey Lime Pita Burger

Preparation Time: 15 minutes

Cook Time: 8 minutes

Serves: 4 servings

Ingredients

1/3 cup breadcrumbs, Italian-seasoned

1/2 cup green onions, chopped

1/2 tsp black pepper, coarsely ground

1 tbsp Moroccan seasoning blend

1 lb. ground turkey

2 (beaten lightly) egg whites, large

1 tbsp olive oil

2 tsps (divided) lime rind, grated

1 1/2 tsps fresh chopped basil

1/2 cup yogurt, plain low-fat

2 cups lettuce, shredded

4 (6") {cut in half} pitas

1/2 cup tomato, diced

Preparation

1. Add the 1 tsp lime rind, ground turkey, egg, black pepper, seasoning blend, breadcrumbs and onions into a bowl and combine well.

2. Form mixture into 8 even (1/4" thick) egg-shaped patties.

3. Add olive oil into a big nonstick skillet over med-high heat.

4. Add patties into the heated oil and cook until well browned for 2 minutes per side.

5. Adjust heat to med-heat and cook for 4 more minutes.

6. Add the basil, yogurt the reserved rind into a bowl and combine.

7. Add 1 tbsp tomato, 1/4 cup lettuce, 1 tbsp basil/yogurt mixture over each half patty.

8. Serve and enjoy.

Nutritional Information/Serving

Calories 426 kcal, Carbs 46.4g, Sodium 776mg, Protein 28.9g, Fat 14g

Swiss Chard with Salmon

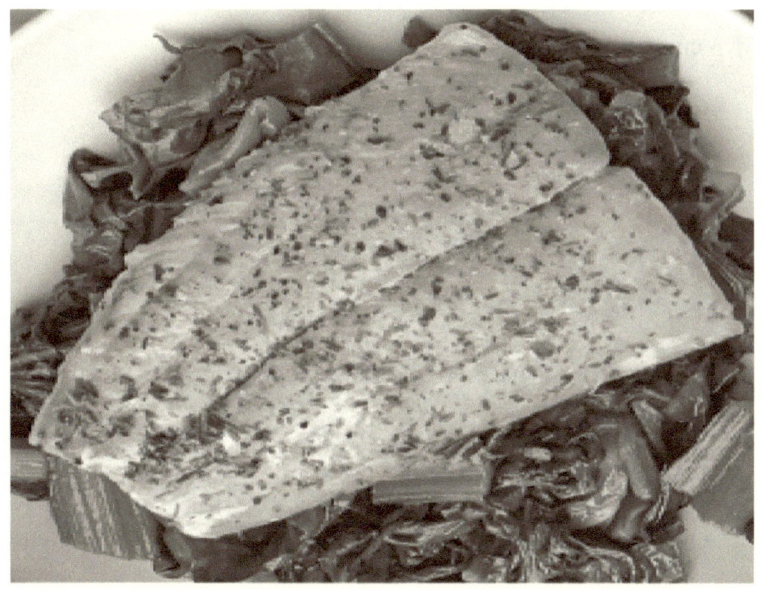

Preparation Time: 10 minutes

Cook Time: 20 minutes

Serves: 4 servings

Ingredients

4 (5 ounces) salmon fillets, skin-on

1/2 cup almond flour

2 1/2 tbsps (divided) olive oil

1 tbsp Dijon mustard

1/2 tsp (divided) black pepper

3/4 tsp (divided) salt

3 (sliced thin) garlic cloves

4 cups Swiss chard stems and leaves, sliced thin

1 tbsp lime juice

1/4 cup dry white wine

1 tbsp fresh rosemary, minced

1 tbsp butter, unsalted

4 lime wedges

Preparation

1. Add almond flour into a flat-bottomed bowl.

2. Coat salmon's flesh side with mustard and lightly press the flesh side into the almond flour dish.

3. Add 1 tbsp olive oil into a big nonstick skillet over med-high heat.

4. Work in two batches, add fillets into the heated pan with the coated side down and cook for 2-3 minutes until just crispy and golden brown.

5. Flip fillets and cook until fillets are well cooked and flesh becomes flaky.

6. Move cooked fillet into a paper towels lined plate.

7. Clean skillet, add 1 tbsp olive oil and repeat process until no fillet remains.

8. Scatter 1/4 tsp pepper and 1/2 tsp salt over cooked fillets until evenly seasoned.

9. Clean the skillet and add 1 1/2 tsp olive oil into the cleaned skillet over med-high heat.

10. Add the chard into the heated skillet and stir cook for 3-4 minutes until just softened.

11. Add garlic into the chard mixture and stir cook for about a minute until aromatic.

12. Add the lime juice and wine into the skillet mixture and cook for about a minute until cooking juices reduces.

13. Add the remaining 1/4 tsp pepper, the remaining 1/4 tsp salt and the butter into the mixture and stir to combine.

14. Split cooked chard into serving platters, topped with chopped rosemary, lime wedges and fish fillets.

15. Serve and enjoy.

Nutritional Information/Serving

Calories 368 kcal, Sodium 591mg, Carbs 6g, Protein 27g, Fat 25g

Basil Turkey Pita

Preparation Time: 15 minutes

Cook Time: 5 minutes

Serves: 4 servings

Ingredients

1 tbsp fresh basil, chopped

2 tsps olive oil

1/2 tsp (divided) salt

1 tsp garlic, minced

1 lb. (cut into 3/4" cubes) turkey breasts, boneless

1/4 tsp black pepper

1 tbsp fresh lime juice

1 1/2 cups seeded cucumber, finely chopped

1 (6 oz.) container yogurt, plain reduced-fat

1/8 tsp black pepper

4 (6") whole wheat pitas

Preparation

1. Add olive oil into a big nonstick skillet over med-high heat.

2. Add the turkey cubes, 1/4 tsp pepper, 1/4 tsp salt, garlic and basil into the heated skillet, toss to combine and cook until well cooked, for about 4 minutes.

3. In the meantime, add yogurt, 1/8 tsp pepper, lime juice, cucumber and 1/4 tsp salt into a bowl and combine.

4. Top 4 whole wheat pitas with even portions of the lamb mixture and dribble with the sauce.

Nutritional Information/Serving

Calories 391 kcal, Sodium 742mg, Carbs 40.8g, Protein 32.7g, Fat 11.5g

Mediterranean Lamb Stew

Preparation Time: 15 minutes

Cook Time: 2 hours 10 minutes

Serves: 6 servings

Ingredients

1 chopped yellow onion, large

Olive oil

6 (peeled and cut into cubes) Yukon gold potatoes

3 (cut into cubes) carrots

3 (coarsely chopped) garlic cloves, large

2 1/2 pounds (trim fat and cut into cubes) leg of American lamb, boneless

1 stick cinnamon

½ cup apricots, dried

1 ½ teaspoon allspice, ground

1 bay leaf

½ teaspoon ginger, ground

1 teaspoon Moroccan spice blend

2 ½ cups beef broth, low-sodium

6 (cut in halves) plum tomatoes from a can

1 (15 ounces) can chickpeas

Preparation

1. Add 2 tablespoons olive oil into a big Dutch oven over med-heat.

2. Heat oil until it shimmers.

Note: don't over heat, oil should not be smoky.

3. Add potatoes, carrots and onions into the hot oil and cook for about 4 minutes.

4. Sprinkle with pepper and salt and add the garlic.

5. Remove veggies from the pot using a slotted spoon, move into a plate and let sit for some minutes.

6. Add extra oil as necessary into the same pot.

7. Add lamb into the oil and brown lamb on every side deeply.

8. Sprinkle pepper and salt over deeply browned lamb.

9. Adjust heat to med-high heat, add the sauteed veggies into the pot with the lamb.

10. Add the spices, bay leaf, cinnamon stick and dried apricots into the pot and stir to combine.

11. Add the broth and plum tomatoes into the pot mixture and bring to boiling for about 5 minutes.

12. Heat up oven to 350°F.

13. Place lid over pot and transfer into the preheated oven and cook for 45 minutes.

14. Check lamb stew to see if broth is needed and add broth as necessary.

15. Cook for 45 more minutes before removing from the oven.

16. Add chickpeas into the pot, place lid over pot, transfer into the oven and cook for 30 more minutes.

17. Take out the pot from the oven and serve at once as desired.

Nutritional Information/Serving

Calories 502 kcal, Protein 43.5g, Total Carbs 65.4g, Sodium 579.7mg, Total Fat 9.7g

Pasta with Lebanese Rice

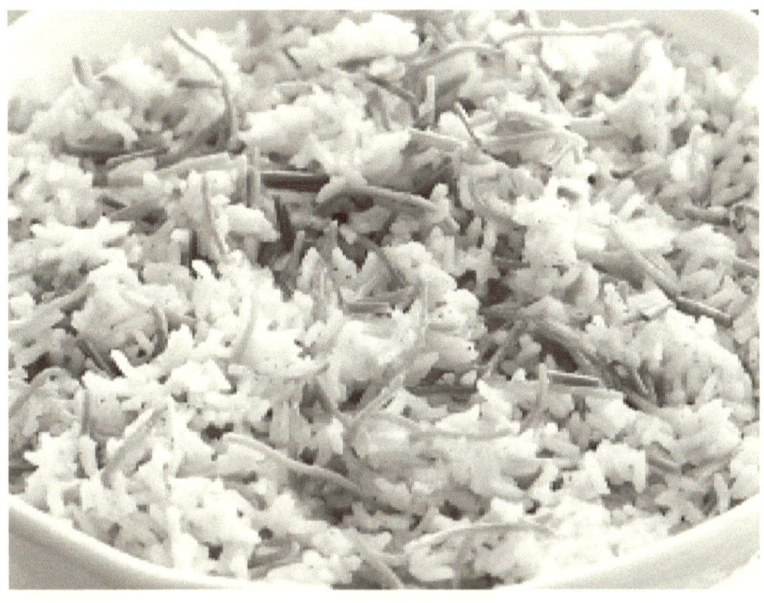

Preparation Time: 15 minutes

Cook Time: 20 minutes

Serves: 6 servings

Ingredients

Water

2 cups (well rinsed) medium grain rice, long grain

2 1/2 tablespoons olive oil

1 cup vermicelli pasta, broken

Salt

Preparation

1. Add just enough water to cover and the rinsed rice into an average bowl.

2. Let rice for 15-20 minutes until soaked.

3. Drain rice well.

Note: Rice should break effortlessly if placed between your index finger and thumb.

4. Add olive oil into an average non-stick pot over med-high heat.

5. Add vermicelli into the hot oil and stir cook until pasta is a fine golden brown and evenly toasted.

Note: Be careful not to burn pasta.

6. Add the rice into the pasta and oil and stir cook until rice is evenly coated with the oil.

7. Sprinkle salt over pasta and rice.

8. Add 3 1/4 cups water into the pot and bring to boiling until water is meaningfully reduced.

9. Adjust heat to low heat and place lid over pot.

10. Cook rice mixture over low heat for 15-20 minutes until wholly cooked.

11. Take rice pot off heat, let sit to cool for 10-15 minutes before uncovering.

12. Remove lid and use a fork to fluff rice.

13. Serve as desired and enjoy.

Nutritional Information/Serving

Calories 331 kcal, Protein 6.4g, Total Carbs 61g, Sodium 0.9mg, Total Fat 5.4g

Lime Scallops with Pasta

Preparation Time: 10 minutes

Cook Time: 18 minutes

Serves: 4 servings

Ingredients

Cooking spray

1 cup orzo, uncooked

1/2 cup onion, chopped

1/2 cup dry white wine

1 cup chicken broth, reduced-sodium, no fat

2 tbsps fresh chopped chives

1/4 tsp oregano, dried

2 tsps olive oil

2 tbsps fresh lime juice

1/4 tsp salt

1 1/2 lbs. sea scallops

1/4 tsp black pepper

Preparation

1. Coat an average saucepan with cooking spray and place over med-high heat.

2. Add onion into the saucepan and cook for 3 minutes.

3. Add oregano, wine, broth and pasta into the onion mixture and bring to boiling.

4. Place lid over saucepan, adjust to low heat and simmer until pasta is al dente and cooking juices is thickened for 15 minutes.

5. Add lime juice and the chopped chives into the pasta mixture and stir to combine.

6. Add olive oil into a big cast iron skillet over med-high heat.

7. Season scallops evenly with pepper and salt.

8. Add seasoned scallops into the skillet and cook until well cooked, for 3 minutes per side.

9. Serve pasta mixture with scallops and enjoy.

Nutritional Information/Serving

Calories 480 kcal, Sodium 875mg, Carbs 45.5g, Protein 60.9g, Fat 5.1g

Pepper Spinach Gnocchi

Preparation Time: 10 minutes

Cook Time: 10 minutes

Serves: 5 servings

Ingredients

1 (5 ounces) baby spinach

1 (16 ounces) potato gnocchi, whole-wheat

3 tbsps (divided) olive oil

6 tablespoons (grated) Parmesan cheese, divided

1/4 cup almonds, smoked

1/2 cup (chopped) roasted red peppers, jarred

1 (torn) baguette slice

1 (chopped) plum tomato

1 garlic clove

2 tbsps sherry vinegar

1/4 tsp red pepper, crushed

1/2 tsp paprika

Preparation

1. Cook potato gnocchi according to instructions on the package.

Tip: exclude oil and salt.

2. Drain water from gnocchi and reserve the cooked gnocchi in the pan.

3. Add 1 tbsp olive oil, 1/4 cup cheese and spinach into the gnocchi, place lid over pan and let sit for 2-3 minutes until spinach is wilted.

4. Toss lightly until combined.

5. Add 2 tbsps olive oil, crushed red pepper, paprika, garlic, vinegar, baguette, tomato and almonds into a food processor and process for about a minute until a smooth consistency is reached.

6. Split gnocchi into serving bowls, and top evenly with cheese and sauce.

Nutritional Information/Serving

Calories 324 kcal, Sodium 590mg, Carbs 34g, Protein 9g, Fat 16g

Crispy Zucchini Pizza

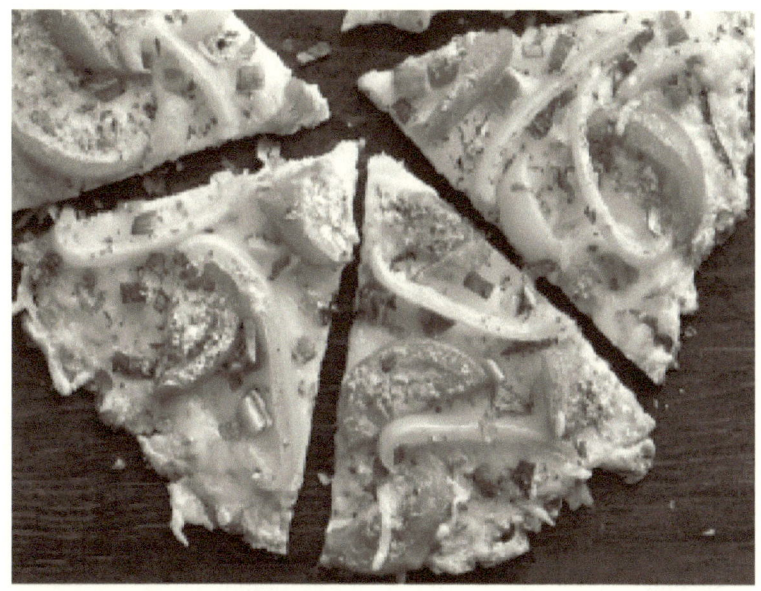

Preparation Time: 10 minutes

Cook Time: 8 minutes

Serves: 4 servings

Ingredients

1 tbsp olive oil

1 tbsp white wine vinegar

1/4 tsp black pepper

1/2 tsp (divided) salt

1 (5 ounces) thin pizza crust, whole-wheat

1 cup zucchini shaved strips

2/3 cup crumbled feta cheese

1/4 cup basil pesto, chilled

1/8 tsp red pepper, crushed

2 (sliced thin) tomatoes, medium

1/2 cup red onion, sliced thin

4 cups mixed greens

1/4 cup fresh chopped oregano

Preparation

1. Heat up oven to 400°F and set rack in the highest position.

2. Add black pepper, 1/4 tsp salt, olive oil and vinegar into an average sized bowl and stir until combined.

3. Add zucchini strips into the vinegar mixture and stir until evenly distributed and let sit for 10 minutes at room temp.

4. In the meantime, transfer the pizza crust to a baking sheet, add basil pesto on top of the crust and spread evenly.

5. Scatter cheese over pizza crust and top with crushed red pepper and tomatoes.

6. Transfer baking sheet into the highest rack of the preheated oven and bake for about 6 minutes until just crisp.

7. Broil pizza for 1-2 minutes on high, until cheese is bubbly.

8. Take off pizza from oven and let sit until cooled for 2 minutes.

9. Add chopped oregano, onion and mixed greens to the zucchini bowl and toss until wholly combined.

10. Add salad mixture over pizza crust and season with the remaining 1/4 tsp salt.

11. Slice pizza into 8 slices and serve at once.

Nutritional Information/Serving

Calories 266 kcal, Sodium 583mg, Carbs 27g, Protein 12g, Fat 17g

Beans Fish Stew

Preparation Time: 5 minutes

Cook Time: 15 minutes

Serves: 4 servings

Ingredients

1 cup onion, chopped

1 tbsp olive oil

1/2 tsp coriander, ground

1 tsp fennel, ground

1 basil sprig

2 crushed garlic cloves

1/4 tsp crushed saffron threads

1/2 tsp fresh orange rind, grated

1 1/2 cups clam juice

1 1/2 cups water

1/8 tsp salt

1 (14.5 oz.) can (undrained) diced tomatoes

1 (14 oz.) can (rinsed and drained) great Northern beans

1 lb. (cut into 2" pieces) flounder fillet

Fresh oregano leaves

Preparation

1. Add olive oil into a big Dutch oven over med-high heat.

2. Add basil sprig, garlic, coriander, fennel and onion into the pot and cook for 5 minutes.

3. Add the saffron and orange rind into the mixture and stir until combined.

4. Add tomatoes, clam juice and water into the pot and bring to boiling.

5. Adjust heat and simmer the tomato mixture for 5 minutes.

6. Add the beans, fish and salt, stir to combine and cook for 5 more minutes.

7. Serve topped with oregano leaves.

Nutritional Information/Serving

Calories 576 kcal, Carbs 94g, Fat 14g, Protein 21g, Sodium 922mg

Spicy Skillet Shrimp

Preparation Time: 10 minutes

Cook Time: 15 minutes

Serves: 4 servings

Ingredients

1 tablespoon flour, all-purpose

1 1/4 pounds (thawed, peeled and deveined) large shrimp

1/2 teaspoon salt

2 teaspoons Spanish paprika, smoked

1/2 teaspoon coriander, ground

1/2 teaspoon pepper

1/4 teaspoon sugar

1/4 teaspoon cayenne

3 tablespoons olive oil

1 tablespoon ghee clarified butter

4 chopped garlic cloves

3 (sliced thin) shallots

1 cup canned diced tomato

1/2 yellow bell pepper and 1/2 green bell pepper, sliced

2 tablespoons dry white wine

1/3 cup preferred broth

1/3 cup chopped cilantro leaves

2 tablespoons fresh lime juice

Preparation

1. Pat dry the shrimp and move into a big bowl.

2. Add sugar, cayenne, coriander, pepper, salt, smoked paprika and flour into the shrimp and toss until evenly covered and coated.

3. Add olive oil and ghee into a big cast iron skillet over med-high heat.

4. Add garlic and shallots into the melted oil and stir cook until aromatic for 2-3 minutes.

Note: Make sure you do not burn the garlic.

5. Add bell peppers into the skillet and cook for about 4 minutes.

6. Toss bell peppers every now and then.

7. Add shrimp into the skillet mixture and cook for 1-2 minutes.

8. Add lime juice, white wine, broth and diced tomatoes into the shrimp mixture and cook until shrimp becomes bright orange, for about 5 minutes.

9. Add fresh chopped cilantro and stir to combine.

10. Serve at once over cooked brown rice, if desired.

Nutritional Information/Serving

Calories 281 kcal, Protein 31.7g, Total Carbs 10.2g, Sodium 244.6mg, Total Fat 13.5g

Flavored Dijon Turkey

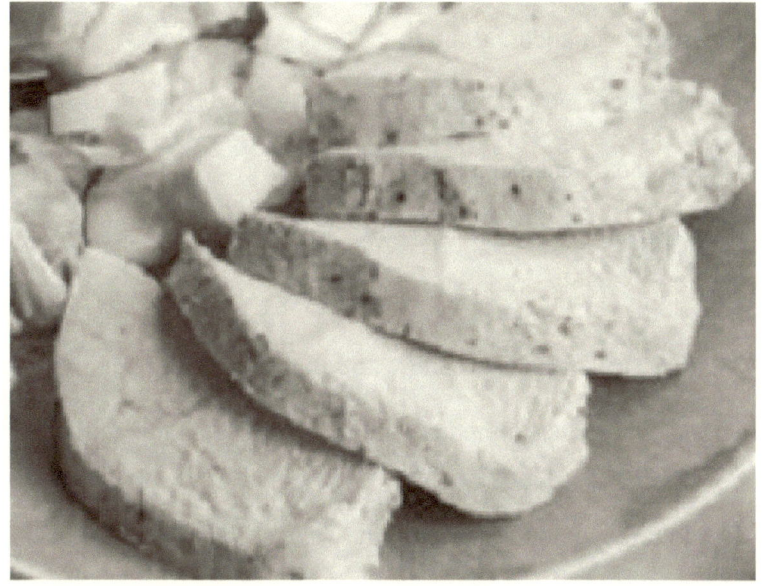

Preparation Time: 5 minutes

Cook Time: 25 minutes

Serves: 8 servings

Ingredients

Salt

1 1/2 pounds (8 pieces) turkey thighs, skinless boneless

1 (cut into large pieces) large yellow onion

Sauce

3 teaspoons Dijon mustard

1/3 cup olive oil

6 minced garlic cloves

2 teaspoons honey

3/4 teaspoon sweet paprika

1 teaspoon coriander, ground

1 pinch salt

1/2 teaspoon black pepper

Preparation

1. Heat up oven to 425°F.

2. Pat dry turkey and sprinkle with salt until all sides are evenly covered.

3. Add every sauce ingredient into a big bowl and mix until well combined.

4. Add turkey into the sauce mixture and stir until wholly coated.

5. Lightly oil a cast iron skillet and add the coated turkey.

6. Add onions and any remaining sauce over turkey in the skillet.

7. Transfer skillet into the prepared oven and bake until an internal temperature of 165°F is reached, and turkey is well cooked for 25-30 minutes.

8. Serve hot, garnished with fresh chopped cilantro.

Nutritional Information/Serving

Calories 284 kcal, Protein 29.8g, Total Carbs 3g, Sodium 454.5mg, Total Fat 16.8g

Greek Salad

Preparation Time: 10 minutes

Cook Time: 0 minutes

Serves: 4 servings

Ingredients

1 (peel partially until strip pattern forms and slice into 1/2" thickness) cucumber

4 (cut into wedges) medium juicy tomatoes

1 (halved and sliced into half-moons) medium red onion

1 (sliced thin) cored green bell pepper

1 pinch salt

Kalamata olives, pitted

1–2 tablespoons red wine vinegar

4 tablespoons olive oil

1/2 tablespoon basil, dried

8 ounces (do not crumble) creamy feta cheese in blocks

Preparation

1. Add cucumber, tomatoes, red onion, bell pepper and olives into a big salad bowl.

2. Lightly sprinkle a pinch of salt over salad and top with red wine vinegar and olive oil.

3. Toss salad mixture until combined.

Tip: Don't over mix.

4. Add feta blocks over salad and sprinkle with dried basil.

5. Serve Greek salad with crusty bread.

Nutritional Information/Serving

Calories 366 kcal, Protein 10.9g, Total Carbs 17.7g, Sodium 1139.1mg, Total Fat 29.5g

SNACKS & NIBBLES

Yummy Butter Cookies

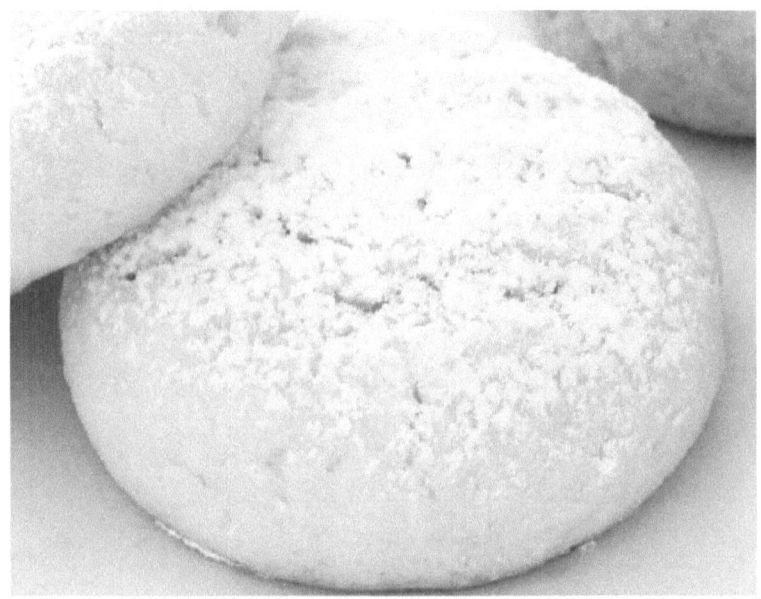

Preparation Time: 10 minutes

Cook Time: 15 minutes

Serves: 35 cookies

Ingredients

1/2 cup (sifted) sugar, powdered

1 cup ghee

2 cups (sifted) flour, all purpose

1/8 scant teaspoon baking powder

Preparation

1. Add ghee into a big bowl and mix on low with an immersion mixer until a whipped consistency is reached.

2. Add the sugar into the whipped ghee and mix on low and adjust speed as necessary to med-sped until a fluffy and smooth consistency is reached.

3. Add 1 cup of all-purpose flour and baking powder into the whipped ghee mixture and knead until flour mixture is fully incorporated with clean hands.

4. Add the reserved 1 cup flour into the mixture and knead one more time until evenly distributed and a very soft dough consistency is reached.

5. Place lid over dough bowl and transfer into a refrigerator until dough is just firmed up, for 20 minutes.

6. Heat up oven to 350ºF.

7. Prepare a parchment paper lined baking sheet.

8. Take out dough from the refrigerator, scoop generous 1/2 tbsps of the dough and form into small dough balls.

9. Press dough ball top lightly.

Note: don't press to flatten.

10. Place dough balls onto the prepared baking sheet and leave about 2-3" distance between each dough ball.

11. Transfer baking sheet into the preheated oven and cook until cookies are slightly colored at the base and firmed up, for about 12-15 minutes.

12. Take out cookies from the oven and let sit until wholly cooled before touching to avoid breaking cookies.

13. Scatter powdered sugar over cooled cookies, serve and dig in.

Nutritional Information/Serving

Calories 82 kcal, Protein 0.7g, Total Carbs 6.9g, Sodium 0.2mg, Total Fat 5.6g

Crispy Italian Biscotti

Preparation Time: 10 minutes

Cook Time: 60 minutes

Serves: 24 cookies

Ingredients

3/4 cup pistachios (salted, shelled, and chopped)

2 eggs

1 teaspoon vanilla extract

3/4 teaspoon green cardamom, ground

1 teaspoon baking powder

2 cups flour, all-purpose

3/4 cup sugar

4 tablespoons (softened) butter, unsalted

Preparation

1. Prepare a parchment paper lined baking sheet.

2. Add baking powder and flour into a small bowl and whisk until combined.

3. Add sugar and butter into a big bowl and mix until beaten and a fluffy light consistency is reached at med-high speed, using a hand mixer.

4. Adjust mixer speed to low.

5. Add an egg into the butter mixture per time and beat lightly on low speed until combined.

6. Repeat process with the remaining egg.

7. Add vanilla extract, cardamom and pistachios into the egg mixture and stir until wholly combined with a spoon.

8. Add the flour mixture into the egg mixture and stir until incorporated.

9. Sprinkle flour over the prepared baking sheet and transfer dough into the prepared baking sheet.

10. Place dough into a refrigerator for 30 minutes.

11. Heat up oven to 350°F with the rack set to center position.

12. Form dough into 12" long with floured hands.

13. Transfer baking sheet into the preheated oven and bake until dough is just golden, for about 25 minutes.

Tip: rotate baking sheet midway while baking.

14. Take baked goods out of the oven and let sit for 10 minutes until cooled.

15. Slice log into 3/8" slices.

16. Transfer sliced biscotti into the baking sheet in a single layer, and leave 1/2" room between each biscotti.

17. Adjust oven temperature to 275°F

18. Bake biscotti until crisp, for 30-35 more minutes.

Note: Flip biscotti midway while cooking.

19. Place baked biscotti on a wire rack and let sit until cooled.

20. Transfer cooled biscotti into a jar with airtight cover, seal and enjoy.

Nutritional Information/Serving

Calories 137 kcal, Protein 1.7g, Total Carbs 14.4g, Sodium 52.3mg, Total Fat 8.2g

Crispy Apple Strudel

Preparation Time: 15 minutes

Cook Time: 35 minutes

Serves: 10 servings

Ingredients

2 tablespoons olive oil

2 teaspoons ghee

1/4 cup brown sugar

3 (peeled, cored and sliced thinly) apples

1/4 teaspoon nutmeg

1 teaspoon cinnamon, ground

2 tablespoons grapefruit juice

1/4 teaspoon cardamom, ground

1/3 cup raisins

1/2 cup walnut hearts, chopped

10 phyllo dough sheets, thawed

Preparation

1. Heat up oven to 375°F.

2. Add olive oil and ghee into a big skillet over med-heat.

3. Add the grapefruit juice, cardamom, nutmeg, cinnamon, brown sugar and slice apples into the heated skillet and stir cook until just cooked, for about 2 minutes.

4. Add the raisins and walnuts into the skillet mixture and stir until evenly distributed.

5. Take skillet off heat and let sit until needed.

6. Drain juices from the skillet into a small bowl, add olive oil, mix and reserve for later use.

7. Prepare a parchment paper lined baking sheet.

8. Arrange 10-12 phyllo sheets on a clean work surface and cover with a towel to prevent drying.

9. Place a sheet of phyllo on the prepared baking sheet and brush with the olive oil/filling juice.

10. Scatter a pinch of brown sugar over the brushed sheets.

11. Repeat process until no phyllo sheet remains.

12. Scoop the skillet mixture (filling) into the center of the phyllo sheets and leave a 2" limit around the edges of each sheet.

13. Brush the edges of the sheet with olive oil and fold over filling until a roll is formed.

14. Brush with extra olive oil and transfer into the preheated oven with the seam side down.

15. Cook until phyllo dough is a fine golden brown, for about 35 minutes.

16. Take baking pan out of the oven and let sit to cool.

17. Top with any remaining raisins or walnut.

18. Slice, serve and dig in.

Nutritional Information/Serving

Calories 132 kcal, Protein 1.5g, Total Carbs 21.3g, Sodium 83.5mg, Total Fat 5g

Nutty Grapefruit Cake

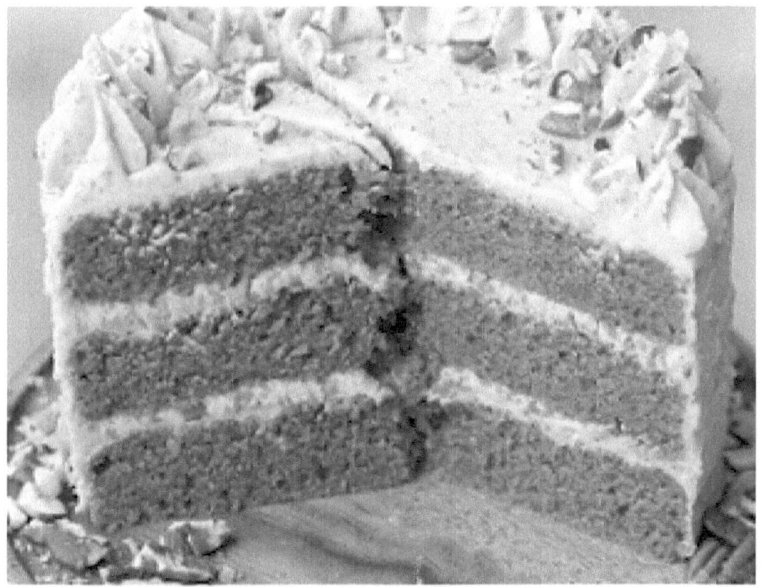

Preparation Time: 10 minutes

Cook Time: 30 minutes

Serves: 15 servings

Ingredients (cake)

1 cup Greek yogurt, plain no-fat

5 eggs, large

5 tablespoons almonds, ground

2 cups sugar, granulated

1 orange, zested

1 lime, zested

1 cup farina, coarse

1 1/4 cup flour, all-purpose

3/4 cup olive oil, plus 1 tablespoon

2 teaspoons baking powder

Syrup

1 1/4 cup honey, runny

1 1 /4 cup salted pistachios, shelled

1 lime, juiced

2 grapefruit, juiced

Preparation

1. Heat up oven to 350°F.

2. Prepare a buttered and floured 9-by-13" baking pan.

Note: Coat evenly with flour after greasing.

3. Add every cake ingredient into a big bowl and whisk until combined.

4. Empty batter into the prepared pan and use a spatula to spread until consistent.

5. Transfer baking pan into the preheated oven and bake until an inserted toothpick comes out clean and cake is golden for 25-30 minutes.

6. Take cake out of the oven and let sit until wholly cooled.

7. In the meantime, place a dry big nonstick skillet over med-heat.

8. Add pistachios into the heated skillet and toast until aromatic.

9. Add honey into the pistachios and stir to combine.

10. Add the lime juice and grapefruit juice and bring to boiling until a fine syrup consistency is reached, for 1-2 minutes.

11. Make holes on the cooled cake top and empty the syrup all over until cake is evenly covered.

12. Slice cake as desired.

Nutritional Information/Serving

Calories 378 kcal, Protein 8g, Total Carbs 66.7g, Sodium 30.1mg, Total Fat 10.3g

Cheesy Grapefruit Cake

Preparation Time: 15 minutes

Cook Time: 45 minutes

Serves: 12 servings

Ingredients

1/2 cup brown sugar

Butter

1 grapefruit, sliced and zested

1 tablespoon water

1 1/2 cup ricotta, part-skim

1 grapefruit, zested

1/2 teaspoon vanilla extract

1/4 cup olive oil, + 2 tablespoons

1 1/2 cup flour, all-purpose

3 eggs, large

3/4 teaspoon kosher salt

2 teaspoons baking powder

3/4 cup sugar, granulated

Dust with

Powdered sugar

Preparation

1. Heat up oven to 325°F.

2. Prepare a liberally buttered 9" baking pan.

3. Line the base of the baking pan with parchment paper.

4. Add water and brown sugar into the prepared pan and stir until a thick paste-like consistency is formed.

5. Spread brown sugar mixture until bottom of the pan is evenly covered.

6. Add the slices of grapefruit into the baking pan over the sugar coating.

7. Add vanilla, olive oil and ricotta into a big bowl and whisk until combined.

8. Whisk in an egg per time into the vanilla mixture until combined.

9. Sift salt, baking powder and flour into the egg/vanilla mixture and whisk until combined.

10. Add the zest of the 2 grapefruits and sugar into a bowl, combine and pour into the flour mixture.

11. Stir mixture again to combine.

12. Spoon and evenly spread batter into the prepared baking pan and transfer into the preheated oven.

13. Bake until an inserted toothpick comes out clean, for 45 minutes until well cooked.

14. Let cake sit until cooled for about 5 minutes before loosening around the edges with a sharp knife.

15. Slice cake and serve as desired.

Nutritional Information/Serving

Calories 179 kcal, Protein 6.2g, Total Carbs 20.1g, Sodium 196.6mg, Total Fat 8.4g

Almond Baklava Rolls

Preparation Time: 15 minutes

Cook Time: 45 minutes

Serves: 20 servings

Ingredients (syrup)

1/2 cup water

3/4 cup sugar

1/2 teaspoon lime juice

1 stick cinnamon

Filling

1/3 cup brown sugar

1 cup lightly toasted almonds

1/4 teaspoon cinnamon, ground

1/4 teaspoon green cardamom, ground

1 pinch salt

1/4 teaspoon cloves, ground

2 tablespoon ghee, melted

Dough

3 tablespoons olive oil

6 phyllo dough sheets

2 tablespoons ghee, melted

Preparation

1. Add cinnamon stick, water and sugar into an average saucepan over high heat.

2. Bring mixture to boiling and stir every now and then until sugar is wholly dissolved.

3. Add lime juice into the mixture, take saucepan from heat, place lid over saucepan and let sit until solid for about 15 minutes.

4. Get rid of the stick of cinnamon and reserve mixture for later use.

5. Add melted ghee, salt, spices, brown sugar and almonds into a blade fitted food processor and process until the filling is rough paste like consistency.

6. Heat up oven to 350°F.

7. Add 2 tbsps melted ghee and 3 tbsps olive oil into a bowl and combine.

8. Arrange 3 phyllo sheets consistently on a flat work surface and brush liberally and evenly with the melted ghee and olive oil mixture.

9. Cut the coated phyllo sheets into 4 even strips, using a sharp knife.

10. Scoop the 1 1/2 tsps almond mixture into each strip along the base edge.

Note: Make sure you leave room on both sides of the almond filling.

11. Roll phyllo strips over filling until a roll is formed.

12. Lightly oil a baking sheet and move roll into the prepared pan.

13. Repeat process until no phyllo sheet remains.

14. Brush melted ghee and olive oil over the arranged baklava rolls and transfer into the preheated oven.

15. Bake until rolls are crisp and browned, for 25-30 minutes.

16. Let sit until cooled and serve with syrup.

Nutritional Information/Serving

Calories 142 kcal, Protein 2g, Total Carbs 15.6g, Sodium 29.9mg, Total Fat 8.5g

Cheese Berry Tart

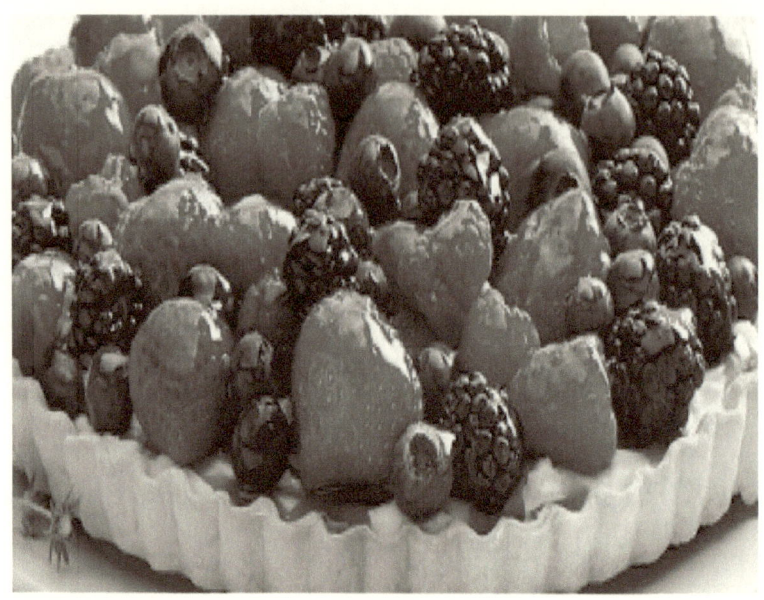

Preparation Time: 15 minutes

Cook Time: 40 minutes

Serves: 8 servings

Ingredients

2 tablespoons sugar

16 ounces (wash and slice thinly) fresh raspberries

1/2 cup olive oil

14 phyllo dough sheets

2–3 tablespoons unsalted pine nuts, crushed

2 tablespoons butter, melted

1 handful oregano leaves, torn

Filling

5 ounces (cut into chunks, at room temp) cream cheese

5 ounces (at room temp) crumbled feta cheese, creamy

2 tablespoons honey

1 tablespoon olive oil

Preparation

1. Heat up oven to 375°F with a rack set at center position.

2. Add sugar and the sliced raspberries into a bowl, toss until combined and move into a colander and let sit.

3. Add honey, olive oil, cream cheese and feta into a blade fitted food processor and process until a smooth paste like consistency is reached.

4. Cautiously roll the phyllo dough sheets on a lightly damp kitchen towel and top with an extra lightly damp towel.

5. Add 2 tbsps butter and 1/2 cup olive oil into a bowl and combine.

6. Casually brush an 11" tart pan with the butter mixture.

7. Arrange 2 phyllo dough sheets into the prepared pan.

Note: The short side of the phyllo sheets should be against the tart pan sides.

8. Coat dough sheets with the butter/olive oil mixture and add 2 extra dough sheets.

9. Coat dough sheet top with the butter mixture.

Note: Arrange the two extra dough sheets in the contrary position until a circle is formed.

10. Repeat process until no dough sheet remains.

Note: Alternate the position of each group of dough sheets.

11. Coat evenly with the butter/olive oil mixture.

12. Fold up the sides of the dough sheets until a rim or edge is formed.

13. Add the honey and cheese mixture into the dough crust, spread and add the crushed pine nuts.

14. Transfer tart pan into a bigger baking sheet.

15. Place baking sheet into the prepared center rack of the preheated oven.

16. Bale until crust is golden brown and crispy and the cheese is melted, for about 15 minutes.

17. Take off heat, let sit until the cheese is cooled and let sit until later.

18. Adorn tart with berries and scatter the torn oregano leaves over tart top.

19. Slice into 8 even pieces and serve.

Nutritional Information/Serving

Calories 445 kcal, Protein 9.4g, Total Carbs 36.5g, Sodium 413.4mg, Total Fat 29.6g

Chocolate Tahini Brownies

Preparation Time: 10 minutes

Cook Time: 30 minutes

Serves: 16 servings

Ingredients

4 ounces dark chocolate chips

4 tablespoons butter, salted

2 eggs, large

3 tablespoons cocoa powder

1 tablespoon vanilla extract

1 cup white sugar, + 2 tablespoons

3/4 cup tahini

1 teaspoon salt

1/3 cup flour, all-purpose

Preparation

1. Heat up oven to 375°F.

2. Place a piece of foil over an 8" square pan with extra foil hanging out of the pan.

3. Place a second piece of foil alternatingly to form a cross with the first foil.

Note: Excess foil should out of the pan on every side.

4. Casually brush aluminum foil with salted butter.

5. Add butter into an average saucepan over med-heat and melt.

6. Take saucepan off heat, add the cocoa and chocolate chips into melted butter and whisk until a smooth consistency is reached.

7. Add salt, vanilla, sugar and eggs into a big bowl and whisk until a lightly thick texture is formed.

8. add tahini into the egg bowl and whisk until combined.

9. Fold in the flour into the egg mixture until just combined.

Note: avoid over stirring.

10. Add the melted butter/chocolate mixture into one half of the flour mixture and stir until evenly distributed.

11. Empty and evenly spread batter into the prepared pan.

12. Transfer square pan into the center rack of the preheated oven and bake until the middle of the brownies remains moist and ends are set.

13. Take out of the oven, let sit to cool for 30 minutes in pan before removing brownies carefully from the pan.

Note: Don't remove foil from brownies yet.

14. Let sit to cool for extra 30 minutes before cutting into 2" square brownies.

15. Serve and dig in.

Nutritional Information/Serving

Calories 226 kcal, Protein 1.8g, Total Carbs 21.3g, Sodium 188.9mg, Total Fat 15.6g

Rice Pudding with Pine Nuts

Preparation Time: 10 minutes

Cook Time: 40 minutes

Serves: 6 servings

Ingredients

1 cup heavy cream

2 cups milk, 2%

2 sticks cinnamon

2 teaspoons vanilla extract

1 cup grain rice, medium

6 whole cloves

1/2 cup water

3 tablespoons sugar

2 tablespoons (at room temp) butter, unsalted

1/3 cup evaporated milk

Serve with

Pine nuts, crushed

Honey

Cinnamon, ground

Preparation

1. Add cloves, cinnamon sticks, vanilla extra, heavy cream and 2% milk into an average saucepan over high heat.

2. Remove saucepan from heat just before the mixture starts to boil.

3. Let heavy cream mixture sit until wholly cool before transferring into a refrigerator until flavors are infused, for 8 hours.

Note: Placing heavy cream in the refrigerator is optional.

4. Remove heavy cream mixture from the refrigerator and let sit for some minutes.

5. Add water, sugar and rice into the heavy cream mixture, place over high heat and bring to boiling.

6. Adjust heat, stir every now and then and simmer for 30-40 minutes.

Note: Add 2 tablespoons of water per time when rice appears dry for even cooking and stir rice mixture every now and then while it cooks until wholly cooked.

7. Remove rice mixture from heat, add the evaporated milk and butter and stir until combined.

8. Get rid of the cloves and cinnamon sticks carefully.

9. Serve as with crushed pine nuts, honey and ground cinnamon.

Nutritional Information/Serving

Calories 383 kcal, Protein 8.4g, Total Carbs 64.3g, Sodium 120.6mg, Total Fat 10.6g

Rich Shortbread Cookies

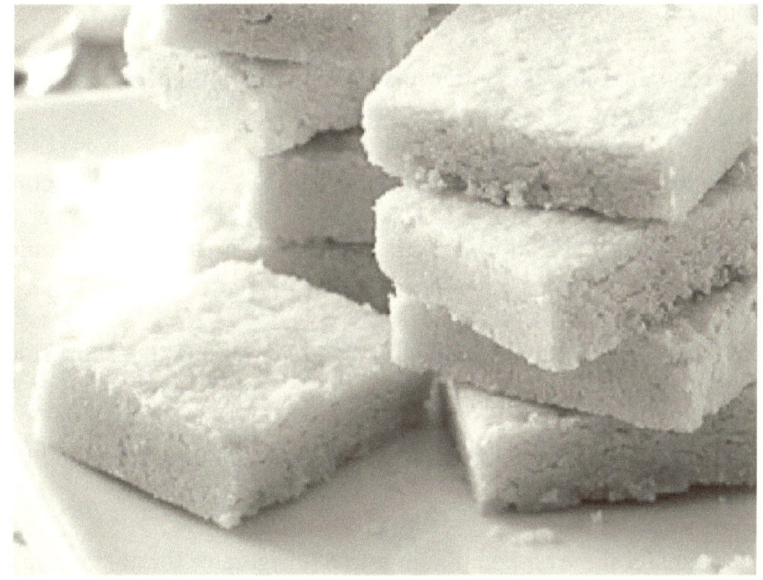

Preparation Time: 15 minutes

Cook Time: 15 minutes

Serves: 24 cookies

Ingredients

1 cup sugar

1 3/4 sticks (at room temp) butter, unsalted

2 cups flour, all-purpose

1 cup tahini paste

1 pinch salt

1 teaspoons baking powder

Preparation

1. Add sugar and butter into a big bowl and mix on med-speed until butter mixture is fluffy and light using a hand mixer.

2. Add tahini into the butter mixture and mix until evenly distributed at med-speed.

3. Add salt, baking powder and flour into a second bowl and combine.

4. Add the flour mixture into the butter mixture and combine until a dough-like consistency is formed.

5. Make dough into a 2" thick log and transfer onto the short side of a big plastic wrap piece.

6. Roll the wrap until dough is wholly and tightly covered and twist at the 2 ends.

7. Transfer the wrapped dough into a refrigerator for an hour or more.

8. Heat up oven to 350°F.

9. Slice the refrigerated dough into about 1/2" rounds and transfer to a very big parchment paper lined baking sheet.

10. Place baking sheet into the preheated oven and bake until cookies are set and browned lightly at the edges, for 15 minutes.

11. Take cookies out of the oven, let sit for about 10 minutes until cooled and move to a cooling rack until wholly cool.

12. Serve and enjoy.

Nutritional Information/Serving

Calories 188 kcal, Protein 1.1g, Total Carbs 18.5g, Sodium 1.4mg, Total Fat 12.5g

Chocolatey Pistachios Stuffed Dates

Preparation Time: 15 minutes

Cook Time: 5 minutes

Serves: 24 servings

Ingredients

24 roasted pistachios, unsalted

24 (make a small hole and remove pits) dates, medjool

1 teaspoon olive oil

1 1/2 cup chocolate chips, semi-sweet

1 tablespoon crushed pine nuts

1 teaspoon cinnamon, ground

Preparation

1. Add a pistachio into the slit of each medjool date and close the opening until pistachio filling is wholly covered.

2. Repeat process with the remaining dates and pistachios, and then let sit in a bowl for later use.

3. Add ground cinnamon, olive oil and chocolate chips into an oven secure bowl.

4. Place bowl over a pot with barely simmering water and stir chocolate mixture continuously until wholly melted.

5. Take off chocolate bowl from heat.

6. Add a date per time into the chocolate mixture and roll until wholly coated.

7. Repeat process until no dates remains uncoated.

8. Transfer coated date onto a parchment paper lined tray in one layer.

9. Sprinkle crushed pine nuts over chocolate coated dates until covered.

10. Transfer tray into a freezer until chocolate is solid for 1 hour.

11. Let sit for 10 minutes at room temp before serving.

Nutritional Information/Serving

Calories 152 kcal, Protein 2g, Total Carbs 27.5g, Sodium 11.2mg, Total Fat 5.4g

Yogurt Parfait with Pumpkin

Preparation Time: 5 minutes

Cook Time: 0 minutes

Serves: 6 servings

Ingredients

1 1/4 cup Greek yogurt, low-fat

2 scant cups pumpkin puree

1 teaspoon vanilla extract

3–4 tablespoons creme fraiche

2 1/2 tablespoon brown sugar

2 tablespoons molasses

1 pinch nutmeg

1 1/2–2 teaspoon cinnamon, ground

Garnish with

Walnuts, chopped

Chocolate chips

Preparation

1. Add every ingredient into a big bowl, excluding the walnuts and chocolate chips.

2. Whisk ingredients until combined and a smooth texture is formed.

3. Check for sweetness by tasting and adjust cinnamon and brown sugar as desired.

4. Mix the mixture again until combined, if necessary.

5. Pour mixture into a small jars, seal and transfer into a refrigerator.

6. Serve, topped with chopped walnuts, chocolate chips and extra dribble of molasses, if desired.

Nutritional Information/Serving

Calories 102 kcal, Protein 0.8g, Total Carbs 15.6g, Sodium 24.5mg, Total Fat 1.5g

Grapefruit Yogurt Crostini

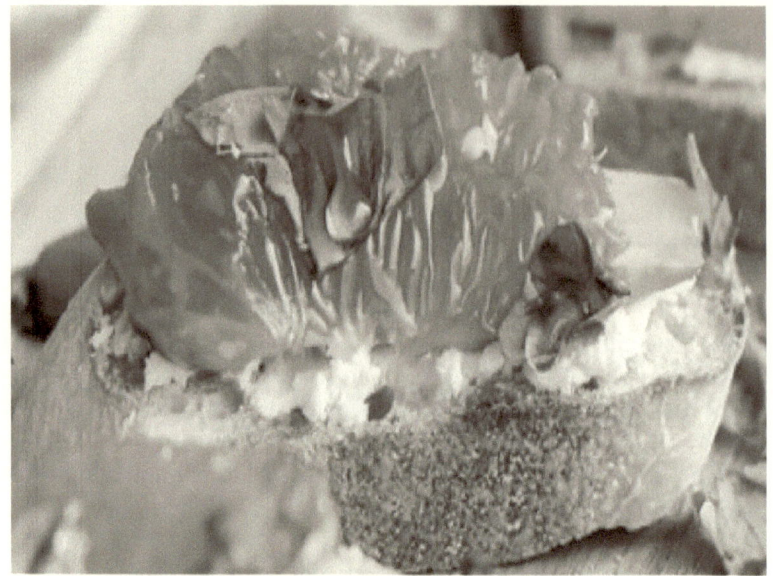

Preparation Time: 10 minutes

Cook Time: 20 minutes

Serves: 10 servings

Ingredients

6 ounces softened cream cheese

1/3 cup Greek yogurt

1/3 cup sugar

1 grapefruit, zested

1 pinch cinnamon, ground

1 pinch nutmeg, ground

3 tablespoons grapefruit juice

3 (cored and thinly sliced into wedges) peaches

1/4 cup walnut halves, coarsely chopped

8–10 (toasted) crostini

Honey

Preparation

1. Add cinnamon, nutmeg, sugar, grapefruit zest, cream cheese and Greek Yogurt into a food process and process until a fluffy and combined consistency is reached.

2. Pour mixture into a bowl, place lid over bowl and refrigerate for 1 hour until needed.

3. Heat up oven to 425°F.

4. Add grapefruit juice and the peaches into a bowl and toss until coated.

5. Lightly pat dry the peaches and transfer to a parchment paper lined baking sheet.

6. Place baking sheet into the preheated oven and bake for 20-25 minutes.

7. Top the toasted crostini with the grapefruit/yogurt mixture and spread evenly.

8. Add the roasted peach slices and chopped walnut over the grapefruit/yogurt mixture and top with honey.

9. Serve and enjoy.

Nutritional Information/Serving

Calories 200 kcal, Protein 4.2g, Total Carbs 28.4g, Sodium 57.3mg, Total Fat 8.5g

Nutty Date Bars

Preparation Time: 15 minutes

Cook Time: 5 minutes

Serves: 16 servings

Ingredients

26 pecan halves

26 (pitted) soft medjool dates, large

3 tablespoons honey

2 (cut into chunks) unsalted butter sticks

1 1/2 cup flour, all-purpose

1 1/2 teaspoons coconut extract

1 cup pine nuts, finely chopped

Preparation

1. Add a pecan half into each date and close opening until pecan filling is wholly covered.

2. Casually grease a small rectangular bowl and add the dates in one layer.

3. Add honey and butter into a small nonstick skillet over med-low heat and melt.

4. Add the coconut extract into the melted butter mixture.

5. Add the flour and stir until combined and stir cook for about 5 minutes until the flour is a fine golden brown in color.

6. Pour the flour mixture into the date mixture until every space is wholly filled and let sit until mixture is set.

7. Add the finely chopped pine nuts over the date cake and press to adhere lightly.

8. Cautiously cut cake into 16 even bars, place lid over bowl and refrigerate for 1 hour.

9. Let sit for 10 minutes at room temperature before you serve.

Nutritional Information/Serving

Calories 587 kcal, Carbs 44g, Fat 44g, Protein 4g, Sodium 14mg

Basil Shortbread Cookies

Preparation Time: 15 minutes

Cook Time: 15 minutes

Serves: 24 servings

Ingredients

1 cup confectioner's sugar

2 cups flour, all-purpose

2–3 teaspoons fresh basil, finely chopped

1/2 cup cranberries, dried

3/4 cup Parmesan cheese, grated

1 pinch salt

2 teaspoons olive oil

226g sticks butter, unsalted

Preparation

1. Add parmesan, salt, basil, cranberries, sugar and flour into a big food processor and process until combined.

2. Add olive oil and butter into the flour mixture and process until a tender dough consistency is reached.

3. Remove dough from food processor cautiously and transfer onto a flat work surface.

4. Roll dough lightly until a log is formed and prepare a long piece of plastic wrap lined foil.

5. Place dough log on the short side of prepared foil and roll until wholly and tightly covered.

6. Twist the 2 ends of the rolled foil and transfer into a refrigerator until solid and chilled.

7. Heat up oven to 375ºF.

8. Cut the chilled log into about 1/2" rounds and transfer into a very large parchment paper lined baking sheet.

9. Place baking sheet into the preheated oven and bake until the cookie edges are lightly brown, for 12-15 minutes.

10. Let cookies sit for some minutes to cool before placing on a cooling rack until completely cool.

11. Serve and enjoy.

Nutritional Information/Serving

Calories 147 kcal, Protein 2g, Total Carbs 14.4g, Sodium 154.6mg, Total Fat 9.1g

Peanut Butter Brownies with Pecan

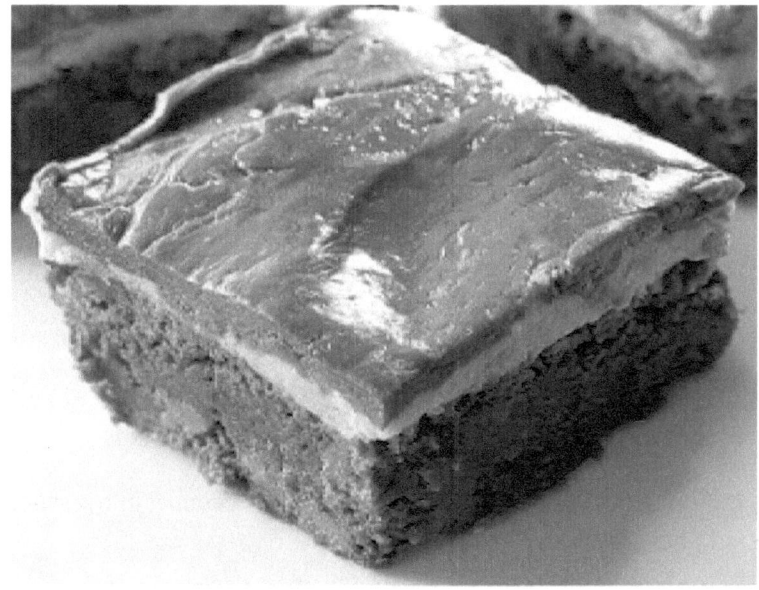

Preparation Time: 10 minutes

Cook Time: 25 minutes

Serves: 8 servings

Ingredients

20 pieces cooking caramel

1 1/2 cup (divided) {coarsely chopped} pecans

2 tablespoons water

1/2 stick (at room temp) butter, unsalted

3/4 cup flour

1 cup peanut butter

1 teaspoon coffee, finely ground

1 teaspoon ground cloves

Sea salt

1 egg

Sauce

2 tablespoons butter

10 pieces cooking caramel

1 tablespoon water

Preparation

1. Heat up oven to 350°F.

2. Add 2 tablespoons water, butter stick and caramel into a saucepan over med-heat and stir cook until melted.

3. Add egg, coffee, ground cloves, flour and peanut butter into a bowl and use a hand mixer to mix until well combined.

4. Add the melted caramel mixture into the flour mixture and mix until combined.

5. Fold in 3/4 cup pecans into the flour/caramel mixture until incorporated.

6. Casually oil an 8-by-8" baking dish and empty the batter into the prepared dish.

7. Transfer baking dish into the preheated oven for 20 minutes until well baked.

8. Take out baking dish from the oven and let sit until cooled.

9. Scatter the remaining pecans and sea salt over brownies.

10. Add 1 tablespoon water, butter and caramel into the same saucepan over med-heat and stir cook until melted.

11. Pour sauce over brownies and slice into 8 even squares.

Nutritional Information/Serving

Calories 721 kcal, Protein 11.9g, Total Carbs 56.2g, Sodium 451.4mg, Total Fat 53.2g

END

Thank you for reading my book.

Bryan Coleman